Ophthalmic Study Guide
for Nurses and Health Professionals

Other Ophthalmology books from M&K:

Eye Emergencies: The practitioner's guide
ISBN: 978-1-905539-08-6 · 2007

Issues in Ophthalmic Practice: Current and future challenges
ISBN: 978-1-905539-17-8 · 2009

Other Health & Social Care books from M&K include:

Routine Blood Results Explained 2/e
ISBN: 978-1-905539-38-3 · 2008

The ECG Workbook
ISBN: 978-1-905539-14-7 · 2008

Arterial Blood Gas Analysis: An easy learning guide
ISBN: 978-1-905539-04-8 · 2008

Nurses and Their Patients: Informing practice through psychodynamic insights
ISBN: 978-1-905539-31-4 · 2009

The Management of COPD in Primary and Secondary Care
ISBN: 978-1-905539-28-4 · 2007

The Clinician's Guide to Chronic Disease Management for Long Term Conditions:
A cognitive-behavioural approach
ISBN: 978-1-905539-15-4 · 2008

Identification and Treatment of Alcohol Dependency
ISBN: 978-1-905539-16-1 · 2008

Perspectives on Death & Dying
ISBN: 978-1-905539-21-5 · 2009

Ophthalmic Study Guide
for Nurses and Health Professionals

Edited by
Dorothy Field
Julie Tillotson
Mandy Macfarlane

The Ophthalmic Study Guide

Dorothy Field, Julie Tillotson and Mandy Macfarlane

ISBN: 978-1-905539-40-6

First published 2009

British Library Cataloguing in Publication Data
A catalogue record for this book is available from the British Library

Notice
Clinical practice and medical knowledge constantly evolve. Standard safety precautions must be followed, but, as knowledge is broadened by research, changes in practice, treatment and drug therapy may become necessary or appropriate. Readers must check the most current product information provided by the manufacturer of each drug to be administered and verify the dosages and correct administration, as well as contraindications. It is the responsibility of the practitioner, utilising the experience and knowledge of the patient, to determine dosages and the best treatment for each individual patient. Any brands mentioned in this book are as examples only and are not endorsed by the Publisher. Neither the publisher nor the authors assume any liability for any injury and/or damage to persons or property arising from this publication.

The Publisher
To contact M&K Publishing write to:
M&K Update Ltd · The Old Bakery · St. John's Street
Keswick · Cumbria CA12 5AS
Tel: 01768 773030 · Fax: 01768 781099
publishing@mkupdate.co.uk
www.mkupdate.co.uk

Designed and typeset in 11pt Usherwood Book by Mary Blood
Illustrations by Mary Blood
Printed in England by Reed's Printers, Penrith

Contents

List of figures

List of tables

About the editors

Dorothy Field RGN, OND, BSc (Hons), MA, EdD recently retired as Senior Lecturer Practitioner (ophthalmic nursing) at Royal Bournemouth and Christchurch Hospitals NHS Foundation Trust and Bournemouth University. She has worked in ophthalmic departments at Bristol, Glasgow and Dublin before spending 23 years in a range of positions in Bournemouth Eye Unit. She is currently employed by Bournemouth eye unit as a 'bank' staff nurse, and is enjoying remaining close to patients and the joys and trials of practice within a busy eye unit. Her most recent publication *Eye Emergencies* was written with Julie Tillotson and published by M&K Update.

Julie Tillotson RGN, OND, BSc (Hons) is currently working as a Nurse Consultant in the Acute Referral Clinic at Bournemouth Eye Unit. She began her ophthalmic nursing career at Moorfields Eye Hospital and then worked as a Nurse Manager at Bournemouth for many years before the lure of clinical practice returned her to the patients. She is known for her innovations to practice, particularly with respect to ophthalmic triage, and the use of computers to enhance safe, efficient, patient-focused management within ophthalmic emergency care.

Mandy Macfarlane RGN, ENB 346, ENB 934, ENB 998/LAPE has a range of ophthalmic experience spanning 20 years. For the last 13 years she has worked as a specialist ophthalmic nurse in acute referral and outpatients where she conducts a number of nurse-led clinics and provides cover for the Nurse Consultant during her absence. She is the educational resource nurse (recently promoted) and clinical assessor for Bournemouth eye unit, where she runs the in-house eye course.

About the contributors

Claire Adams RGN, OND has been working in ophthalmology since 1987. She has worked in various ophthalmic departments in Wolverhampton and Salisbury before settling at Bournemouth Eye Hospital. She is currently employed as a Senior Staff Nurse in the Cataract Clinic, where she involves herself in pre-assessment and postoperative cataract follow-up clinics. She is currently undertaking a BSc in Applied Health Studies.

Sue Cox SRN, BA (Hons), ENB 346 qualified in 1976. After working in Theatres and in Gynaecology she joined Bournemouth Eye Unit in 1997. She is currently working in the Acute Referral Clinic as a Senior Staff Nurse.

Lynn Ring RGN, RNLD, ENB 346 & 998, BSc (Hons) works in the ophthalmic outpatient accident and emergency unit at Epsom and St Helier University Hospitals NHS Trust. She has worked as an ophthalmic nurse since the early 1990s as a staff nurse, ward sister and matron and now is a nurse specialist. She has achieved a number of clinical competencies supported by degree and master's level education and works within the glaucoma service managing her own caseload and in the accident and emergency unit seeing all types of emergency patients.

Acknowledgements

The following staff have also contributed expert knowledge to this publication: Anita Balestrini, Pauline Haley, Anne-Marie Lacey, Linda Martin, Non Mathews, Faith Ooi, Marion Owen, Anthea Reid, Yvonne Walker and the wider staff in every speciality at Bournemouth Eye Unit. All photographs are courtesy of Samantha Hartley, Ophthalmic Photographer, Royal Bournemouth Hospital, UK. I would also like to thank Maria Hampshire at Shoreline BioMedical for her editorial expertise.

Preface

Multiprofessional care of the ophthalmic patient

Over recent years, an increasing variety of professionals have been involved in the care of ophthalmic patients. The aim underlying the changes of the last 20 years has been to provide an efficient, high-quality and cost-effective service to patients, which utilises the skills of the multidisciplinary ophthalmic team. The move to more day-case ophthalmic surgery released ophthalmic nurses to participate in the more complex preparation of patients for very short stays. The increased patient turnover for example, required nurses, orthoptists, technicians and optometrists to expand their skills to participate in using a range of measurement equipment so that accurate intraocular lens measurements could be provided to ophthalmic surgeons. Nurses and optometrists are increasingly managing their own patient groups in clinics under protocols so that consultant ophthalmologists can supervise their burgeoning caseloads.

Research in 2006 by Czuber-Dochan, Waterman and Waterman revealed that this expansion of nursing roles is set against a background of an increasing shortage in expert ophthalmic nursing. They revealed a downward trend in the number of nurses working in ophthalmology, alongside an expansion of technology that is stimulating a demand for more advanced levels of ophthalmic clinical nursing practice. Over the period of the three surveys (Waterman *et al.*, 1995; Waterman and Waterman, 1999) there has been a decline in the numbers of nurses holding skills-based ophthalmic nursing courses.

Furthermore, the more recent Czuber-Dochan *et al.* (2006) study revealed that out of three nurse consultants surveyed only two claimed to have an ophthalmic qualification, and of 259 nurses working at an advanced level only 83.4% stated they had an ophthalmic qualification. Most ophthalmic nursing qualifications are now ophthalmic modules at university academic level H. While this does denote a deeper level of academic learning, the theoretical assessments are, of necessity for 20 credit units, often very narrowly focused to ensure the demonstration of depth of knowledge.

The authors have produced this *Ophthalmic Study Guide* to provide the opportunity for nurses or other health professionals new to ophthalmology (e.g. operating department practitioners who work in ophthalmic perioperative practice settings) to develop useful, basic knowledge quickly. It will also help individuals to develop a broad, practical knowledge base prior to undertaking focused higher ophthalmic education.

In an investigation into the development of advanced practice roles in ophthalmic nursing, Marsden and Shaw (2007) did not record whether the nurses they reported on had undertaken any recognised ophthalmic courses or structured studies prior to beginning their specialised practice. They do note, however, that 'services must consider the need for education as well as training for new roles.'

In 1995, Sweet and Norman reviewed the 'doctor–nurse game', a pattern of interaction from the 1960s whereby nurses learned to show initiative and offer advice while appearing to defer passively to the doctor's authority. By 1988, Hughes' research in a UK casualty department (Hughes, 1988) surmised that the traditional dominant/subservient model was vanishing, with nurses' work focusing more on diagnosis and treatment, being largely responsible for the categorisation of patients, history taking and often indicating the likely course of treatment before the patient was seen by a doctor for formal diagnosis. Currently, experienced ophthalmic nurses, having received adequate education and practice, are taking major roles in terms of patient assessment, minor surgery, acute referral clinics and prescribing.

This *Study Guide* cannot be considered to be a substitute for more formal, assessed education and training for role expansion, but can be considered in terms of being a 'skills escalator' in that those who make good use of its contents and use the *To Do* boxes to reflect on and research their practices should be able to develop their basic knowledge and skills in practice more quickly, and develop the habit of self-assessment and self-directed learning. The simple questions at the end of many chapters can be used for self-testing, or as a basis for questions that mentors might ask. Indeed, Edmond (2001) states the significance of exploring the nature of professional practice itself, and warns of the danger of disregarding the importance of the practice context because of an assumption that practice is 'easily picked up' once the individual is qualified. She also goes on to comment on the 'pivotal issue' regarding availability of staff nurse mentors. It is hoped that the guidance that follows will enable new staff members and their mentors to enjoy a highly productive educational relationship.

The content of this book has deliberately been restricted to "the basics" in terms of the areas chosen, although they are all covered in reasonable depth. Students are encouraged to use the skills checklists in Appendix 1 to document their personal progress and validate their developing practice. Partially completed checklists will be useful evidence for annual appraisals.

Did you know?

According to the Federation of Domestic and Ophthalmic and Dispensing Opticians, Domiciliary Eyecare Committee and College of Optometrists (2007):

- 4 million people over the age of 60 in the UK do not have regular sight tests (even though they are entitled to free eye examinations).
- 1.7 million people over the age of 65 in the UK have significant sight loss; 85% of blind and partially sighted people are over 65 years old. Glaucoma, age-related macular degeneration and diabetic retinopathy must be detected early in order to avoid or minimise sight loss.
- 270,000 people over the age of 75 in the UK experience unnecessary sight loss because they do not wear spectacles or because they wear outdated spectacles.
- 89,500 falls requiring hospital treatment in the UK happen because of some visual impairment (costing the NHS nearly £300 million) and 14,000 people die every year as a result of osteoporotic hip fractures. Some studies that consider visual impairment as part of their falls reduction plan have shown as much as a 14% drop in the number of falls.

References

Czuber-Dochan, W., Waterman, C. and Waterman, H. (2006). Atrophy and anarchy: Third national survey of nursing skill-mix and advanced nursing practice in ophthalmology. *Journal of Clinical Nursing*, 15, 1480–88.

Edmond, C. (2001). A new paradigm for practice education. *Nurse Education Today*, 21, 251–59.

Federation of Domestic and Ophthalmic and Dispensing Opticians, Domiciliary Eyecare Committee and College of Optometrists (2007). *A Fundamental Right to Sight*. London: Domiciliary Eye Care Committee.

Hughes, D. (1988). When Nurse knows best. Some aspects of nurse–doctor interaction in a casualty department. *Sociology of Health and Illness*, 10(1), 1–22.

Marsden, J. and Shaw, M. (2007). The development of advanced practice roles in ophthalmic nursing. *Practice Development in Health Care*, 6(2), 119–30.

Sweet, S. and Norman, I. (1995). The nurse–doctor relationship: a selective literature review. *Journal of Advanced Nursing*, 22, 165–70.

Waterman, H. and Waterman, C. (1999). Trends in ophthalmology services, nursing skill mix and education. Second National Survey. *Journal of Advanced Nursing*, 30, 94–49.

Waterman, H., Hope, K., Beed, P., *et al.* (1995). Nature of ophthalmic services and the education and qualifications of nurses who care for patients: a national survey. *Journal of Advanced Nursing*, 22, 779–84.

More about this book

We have used a flag system within some chapters of this book. Flag symbols have been placed within the text to highlight the diagnostic significance of symptoms described in particular contexts.

 A red flag indicates a significant, potentially urgent symptom or fragment of significant knowledge.

 An amber flag indicates a symptom that requires careful evaluation, or a fragment of useful information.

 A mass of excellent information is now available at the click of a button. A wide range of useful websites and electronic libraries have been explored during the writing of this book, and all are clearly marked by the mouse icon.

Many well-referenced, peer-reviewed papers are also freely available, and these resources are also quoted so that you can, if you wish, read many of the original articles. In some areas of the book where specific online material can help you with the set activities, a web resource is indicated to start you on your way.

All the reference lists have been divided into print-based and web-based information to make it clear where there is an immediate opportunity to read an academic paper in full, or to look at a well-illustrated or interactive web resource.

The National Library for Health, cited extensively throughout has become NHS Evidence Health Information Resources. National Library for Health still appears on Google searches. The web address is the same.

Chapter 1

Information for students and mentors

Dorothy Field

The purpose of this book is to guide your learning in the clinical environment. It encourages an extensive use of the internet, so that you can watch animated models of how conditions develop and are treated, and points to some films of surgical procedures. This chapter explains how the guide may be used in the clinical setting, and how a personal portfolio may be used by mentor, student and manager as evidence of personal development for the Knowledge and Skills Framework (KSF). You are reminded that the ophthalmic nursing competencies of the Royal College of Nursing (RCN, 2005) or the Scottish Professional Development Portfolio's *Route to Enhanced Competency in Ophthalmic Nursing* (NHS Scotland, 2002) may be used within a folder of evidence to show how you are meeting your KSF job description.

 If you are not a nurse, it is recommended that you visit the website of the Association of Health Professionals in Ophthalmology (AHPO) and relate your studies to the Ophthalmic and Visual Science National Occupational Standards by checking their Ophthalmic and Visual Standards. These standards relate directly to the KSF Health and Wellbeing (HWB) standards.

By helping you understand some of the theoretical background in the care of ophthalmic patients it is expected that you will be able to more rapidly progress your competence within practice. The knowledge and skills obtained will provide a useful foundation to subsequent academic study and development of specialist practice.

Change, with the requirement to help more patients every year, using equipment that is continually evolving requires new methods of learning and working and is the greatest challenge of the 21st century. Indeed Bill Clinton, former President of the USA, stated in 1998 that the volume of available knowledge was doubling every 5 years. He acknowledged that innovations like human genome research meant that problems could be solved within a matter of days rather than years as had been the case before he took office. He estimated that the worldwide web was growing by around 65,000 web sites every single hour in the late 1990s, but when he took office there were only 50 web sites. The web had started out as the province of just a handful of physicists, in fact, as part of a government research project in the Defence Department. After this basic research, which got the system up and running, the worldwide web soon become the fastest growing organ of human interaction in history.

Lifelong learning

Whether you are a registered nurse, a healthcare assistant or a member of another healthcare profession, a lifelong approach to learning is increasingly necessary due to the speed of change in knowledge and technical developments.

On its website, the *Nursing and Midwifery Council* states that 'as the pace of change in the delivery of health care and the public's expectations of registered practitioners continue to increase, the principles and values of lifelong learning are increasingly important to all registered practitioners'.

To work well, a lifelong approach to learning needs to exist primarily as part of one's attitude to life in general. Secondly, it needs to be adopted within working teams, where questions are welcomed and information and skills are readily shared. Finally, lifelong learning requires 'top down' support from the employer, including availability of textbooks and access to the internet within the clinical setting, a good annual appraisal system with six-monthly 'follow-ups' on progress towards objectives and realistic training and educational plans for staff.

Getting yourself organised to learn about the eye

You will need:

A *mentor*: This person should be an experienced professional, preferably with an ophthalmic qualification. Choose someone you like, who is respected for his or her excellent clinical practice. If you are a nurse, your mentor should have completed a recognised ophthalmic nursing course or be academically competent in ophthalmic theory and practice as applied to nursing.

Two folders: The first is a *professional portfolio* in which you will store 'summary' information to show how you are meeting the main headings of your Knowledge and Skills (KSF) job description. The RCN Ophthalmic Competencies (2005) or AHPO Occupational Standards can help you to demonstrate that you are meeting your job description by developing your ophthalmic competency. The second is a *personal folder* for you to store your personal notes on the tasks you have been set as you study this course. This will enable you to look over what you have achieved, and discuss your progress with your mentor.

Access to the internet: If you do not have access at home, it may be possible to check some facts on a computer at work. The addresses of some particularly useful sites are provided throughout this study guide.

Access to the National Library for Health: Particularly useful for academic papers, health information and Cochrane Reviews of research evidence if you are doing a general internet search on a subject. Academic papers inaccessible to the general public are listed.

Register with the *National Library of Health* website so that you can search for research evidence at work and at home. If you have any problems, ask your hospital librarian to set up the account for you and to demonstrate how to use it most effectively.

Competence

The aim of this study guide is professional competence. The Royal College of Nursing (RCN, 2005) states that the current UK vocational movement places emphasis on competence to do the job – not on the person – and on minimum standards to do the job rather than superior performance. The RCN comment that this kind of approach to competence emphasises workplace performance instead of underpinning knowledge. The RCN prefer Roach's approach (Roach, 1992), which suggests that competence is the state of having the knowledge, judgement, skills, energy, experience and motivation required to respond adequately to the demands of one's professional responsibilities.

Clearly, competent practice also requires an evidential base. Sackett *et al.* (1996) offer a medical definition of an evidence-based approach to practice, which is increasingly applicable to nursing. They see this approach as the conscientious, explicit and judicious use of current best evidence in making decisions about the care of individual patients. It involves integrating individual clinical expertise with the best available external clinical evidence from systematic research. Sackett *et al.* define clinical expertise as the professional judgements that individual clinicians acquire through clinical experience and clinical practice.

Bearing this in mind, together with your mentor, you must seek to achieve the higher levels of Bloom's taxonomy (Bloom *et al.*, 1956) in terms of your cognitive, affective and psychomotor development within ophthalmology (a taxonomy is a technical term for a list that systematically classifies, ranks or prioritises concepts). Check this out on the internet. As you are beginning to see, learning begins at the basic level of just knowing about something and, in the committed individual, may progress as far as re-designing the manner in which an ophthalmic service is managed (for example, in terms of better patient outcomes, motivated staff, increased efficiency or better use of resources). This is all about developing the HOTS for ophthalmology – otherwise known as Higher Order Thinking Skills!

Staying up to date

When you have finished your studies with this guide, it is a good idea to keep your eyes open for other ophthalmic textbooks. Aim to purchase one new book per year. In this way, you will have your own little resource library at home so that you can build on your understanding of more complex conditions, and keep your knowledge up-to-date. It is a good idea throughout your working life if after an 'early' duty you spend just 10 minutes at home looking up something you did not understand. If you decide to study a suitable university ophthalmic unit, you will be well prepared for higher-level studies, both in terms of having good knowledge as well as your own study materials.

The National Health Service Knowledge and Skills Framework

The KSF is the key to the pay system of the NHS.

Check the NHS website for their KSF core dimensions, levels and indicators. Progression through the 'gateways' of your pay band will be dependent on you being able to provide enough evidence at your appraisal to show that you have met your personal development plan for the year. You can probably find copies of KSF linked appraisal forms on your Trust's intranet.

> The ideal way to prepare for your annual KSF appraisal is by collecting material about your learning in your professional portfolio between one appraisal and the next.
>
> ● You can progress at your own rate.
>
> ● It can be specific to ophthalmology.
>
> ● It can meet PREP (post-registration experience and practice) requirements of the Nursing and Midwifery Council.

Visit the website of the Nursing and Midwifery Council where you can read the *PREP Handbook*.

Suggestions for preparing your professional portfolio

Obtain a folder and buy a pack of ten dividers. This portfolio will differ from previous portfolios because it must contain up-to-date evidence – it should not be more than a year old. Work on producing your evidence for assessment and place it in your professional portfolio in the following sections:

Section 1: Write a very short but current summary CV, just about a page long. Date and sign it to show that it is up-to-date.

Section 2: Make a truthful self-appraisal of your personal strengths, weaknesses, opportunities and threats (SWOT). Then date it and sign it. It will probably give you some insight into areas of your nursing practice that you need to develop or modify.

Section 3: Make a personal action plan for the year to come, taking into account what you found out about yourself by doing the SWOT self-appraisal. Date it and sign it. This could include beginning to work your way through the RCN's ophthalmic competencies and learning all the diagrams in this book so that you can understand more fully patients' eye conditions and the patient-focused clinical examinations, notes and conversations of professional colleagues. It could also include some of the skills you will need to carry out competently in practice. Make a new plan every year and make achievable goals, bearing in mind the level of support you can expect at work, as well as patient throughput and demands on your personal life.

You can find out more about ophthalmic competencies on the websites of the Royal College of Nursing or the Association of Health Professionals in Ophthalmology.

Section 4: This is where you will keep your Agenda for Change job description so that it is readily available for reference.

Section 5: It will be useful to keep a short overview of the NHS Knowledge and Skills Framework here.

You can use the other numbered sections of your professional portfolio (sections 5 to 10) to demonstrate that you are meeting the core requirements of the NHS Knowledge and Skills Framework. Your job description will show you what other sub-dimensions you need to meet. You will probably find that they will all fit in with the core requirements below.

- Communication.
- Personal and people development.
- Health, safety and security.
- Service improvement.
- Quality.
- Equality and diversity.

You will have to study your RCN Ophthalmic Competencies or Ophthalmic Vocational Standards (OVS) or the Scottish route to enhanced competence in ophthalmic nursing and decide how you are going to fit the evidence that you will be providing around the KSF core and specific requirements and collect the evidence you will require. The RCN publication on competencies (RCN, 2005) gives you many examples of types of evidence that could be used. The OVS and Scottish ophthalmic competencies also provide good clinical focus for development. Doubtless your work will be a mixture of short reflective studies, witness statements and signed evidence of skills development.

References and further reading

Bloom, B., Englehart, M., Furst, E., Hill, W. and Krathwohl, D. (1956). *Taxonomy of Educational Objectives: The Classification of Educational Goals. Handbook I: Cognitive Domain*. New York, Toronto: Longmans Green.

Clinton B. (1998). Remarks by the US President to the National Association of Attorneys General at Washington Court Hotel, 12 March 1998. Washington DC: The White House Press Secretary Office.

NHS Scotland (2002). *Scottish Professional Development Portfolio – A Route to Enhanced Competency in Ophthalmic Nursing*. Edinburgh: NHS Education for Scotland.

Roach, M. (1992). *The Human Act of Caring: A Blueprint for the Health Professions*. Ottawa: Canadian Hospitals Association Press.

Royal College of Nursing Ophthalmic Forum (2005). *Competencies: An Integrated Career and Competency Framework for Ophthalmic Nurses*. London: RCN.

Sackett, D., Rosenberg, W., Muir Gray, J., Haynes, R. B. and Richardson, W. S. (1996). Evidence based medicine: What it is and what it isn't. *British Medical Journal* 312, 71–72.

Useful web resources

Association of Health Professionals in Ophthalmology (AHPO)
http://www.ahpo.org/

Institute of Virtual Training Suites: Internet Detective
http://www.vts.intute.ac.uk/detective/index
A service for universities and colleges offering web-based tutorials teaching internet research skills

National Health Service
http://www.dh.gov.uk/en/index.htm

Scottish Professional Development Portfolio (Ophthalmic Nursing)
http://www.scotland.gov.uk/Topics/Health/NHS-Scotland/

National Library for Health
http://www.library.nhs.uk/rss/

Nursing and Midwifery Council
http://www.nmc-uk.org/

Basic anatomy and physiology of the eye

Dorothy Field

Basic knowledge of anatomy and physiology of the eye is essential if we are to identify and use the correct names for the various structures and understand eye disorders. Ophthalmic professionals need to have a reasonable grasp of the correct vocabulary to create accurate documentation and make precise verbal communications. Always look up everything as it crops up in practice. In this way, learning will become a habit that makes clinical work interesting – not a chore.

The eye as a whole

You need to memorise all the basic diagrams in this chapter. Some people find that drawing the diagram out on a page of their personal folder helps them to learn its main features, helping them remember where each part is and the name of each structure without prompting. When examining the eye, it is normal to start from the outside and work inwards, so this is the most logical way to study the anatomy (Fig. 2.1).

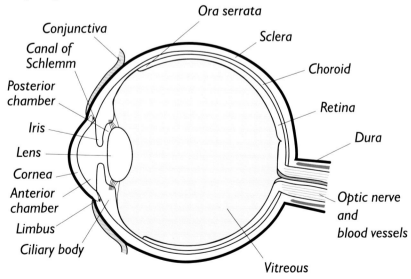

Figure 2.1 *The eye.*

The bony orbit is commonly described as being pyramid shaped, with the highest point at the optic foramen (a passage through a bone generally for nerves and blood vessels to pass through) in the sphenoid bone, which provides the entrance to the optic canal. The optic canal carries the optic nerve, the ophthalmic artery and sympathetic nerve fibres from the carotid plexus. A fracture at or near the optic canal may cause damage to the optic nerve, resulting in visual loss.

The superior orbital fissure lies between the lesser and greater wings of the sphenoid bone. Through this foramen pass the oculomotor, trochlear and abducens nerves and the ophthalmic division of the trigeminal nerve. The superior ophthalmic vein leaves the orbit through the upper part of the superior orbital fissure.

The greater wing of the sphenoid bone and the orbital plate of the maxillary bone form the inferior orbital fissure. This transmits the maxillary division of the orbital branch of the trigeminal nerve and the inferior ophthalmic vein.

The bony margins of the orbit provide general protection to the eye from impact with larger objects, such as footballs. Smaller objects like stones and squash balls are likely to cause more damage. Fractures of the orbital margin generally cause no lasting problems with the eye. The orbital floor is very thin and may 'blow out' into the maxillary sinus with a blunt eye injury such as that sustained by impact with a fist or tennis ball. The orbital contents, including the inferior rectus and inferior oblique muscles, may get trapped in the fracture site, causing restriction of eye movements and double vision (diplopia) in some positions of gaze. A fracture into the thin ethmoid bone medially may be associated with subcutaneous emphysema of the eyelids when the patient blows his or her nose.

Blood supply to the eye and orbit

Both the arterial blood supply to and the venous drainage from the orbit are located within the cavernous sinus. The ocular nerve, trochlear nerve, ophthalmic nerve, abducent nerve and maxillary nerve also pass through this sinus. This is of particular significance if a patient develops orbital cellulitis, because without prompt antibiotic treatment there is a danger of infection passing back into the cavernous sinus.

The eyelids

The edge of each eyelid is called the eyelid margin. The space between the two eyelids when the eyes are open is called the palpaebral fissure. The tiny openings to the tear drainage system in the nasal corners of each eye are called the lacrimal puncta (plural) or punctum (one). The corners of the eyelids are called the medial canthus (nearest the nose) and the lateral canthus (at the temple). The powerful muscle that closes the eyelids is called the orbicularis oculi, which encircles each eye. This is very significant when a person has a painful eye injury such as a chemical burn to the eye – it is very hard to get the eye open to wash the chemical out due to the reflex spasm of this muscle.

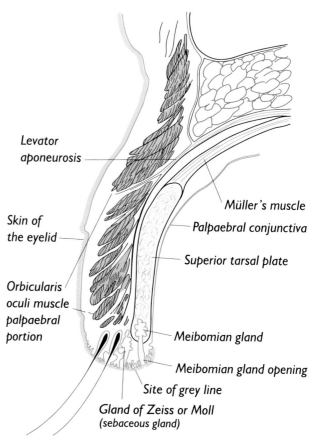

Figure 2.2 *The eyelid.*

The muscles responsible for keeping the upper eyelids open are the levator muscle, Muller's muscle and the frontalis muscle of the brow. Each eyelid is lined by thin cartilage, called *tarsal plates*, which give shape and strength to the lids and provide protection to the eye.

The eyelids are lined with conjunctiva (see Fig.2.2). The eyelid is key to understanding many of the external eye disorders, so it is important to learn the structure of the eyelid.

To do ...

Think about the eyelids carefully and list their main functions in your folder. There are many potential problems with malfunctioning eyelids. With the help of colleagues, start to make a list of all the eyelid problems you can find under the following headings:

- Problems with eyelid closure.
- Problems with eyelid opening.
- Infections and inflammations.
- Eyelash problems.

The lacrimal apparatus

The *lacrimal gland* is a small, almond-shaped gland situated beneath the conjunctiva, in the lacrimal fossa of the orbital bones on the upper, outer side of each orbit. Its outline can be seen under the skin of emaciated people. The lacrimal gland has several short ducts that open into the upper conjunctival fornix, and its sensory nerve supply comes from the lacrimal nerve, a branch of the ophthalmic division of the trigeminal nerve.

As you can see from Fig. 2.3 the *tear film* is composed of three layers. The inner mucin layer is secreted by goblet cells in the conjunctiva, and lies over the endothelial surface of the cornea. Its complex structure is critical for holding the aqueous (watery) layer of the tears on the front of the eye. The aqueous layer is the thickest, and keeps the surface of the eye healthily moist and clean. The oily layer, produced by the meibomian glands (see Fig. 2.2) further assists in holding the aqueous layer of the tears on the front of the eye and inhibits evaporation of the tear film. A healthy tear film is critical to the health of the surface of the eye, and blocked meibomian glands are a significant cause of problems with the tear film.

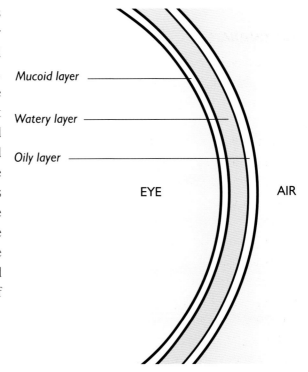

Figure 2.3 *The tear film.*

To do ...

Make notes on the causes of dry eyes.

Good areas for investigation are Marsden (2008) and the Patient UK and BBC Health websites. Be aware, however, that many of the internet sites you may look at are commercial and may be promoting particular products, or may belong to special interest groups who are keen to promote particular points of view.

Diagnosis of dry eyes

Make notes on Schirmer's test. This is described in Chapter 13 but your notes should be based on one you have done yourself! What is the normal result for this test? How reliable is it in practice? Fluorescein break-up time is a frequently used test for dry eye. How reliable is it? Have a look at Moore *et al.* (2009) who discuss the accuracy of these and other dry eye tests in detail. Do remember, however, that *participating* in these examinations, gaining information from experienced colleagues and examining many patients are equally important.

Treatment of dry eyes

See the section in the latest *British National Formulary* on tear deficiency and ocular lubricants. Different groups of 'artificial tears' are used for the differing problems with the tear film.

Tear production

Tear production is of three main types:

Basal tears: These are produced all the time, at a constant rate, to lubricate the front of the cornea and the conjunctiva covering the eyeball and lining the eyelids. Most of the middle aqueous layer of basal tear film is produced by the minor accessory glands of Krause and Wolfring located in the superior fornix, plus some secretions from the lacrimal gland.

Reflex tears: These are secreted by the lacrimal gland in response to irritation produced by a foreign body, allergen or chemical.

Psychogenic tears: These are believed to be unique to humans (unless of course crocodiles really do cry!) and they flow when the crying process is triggered in a healthy person in response to strong emotion.

Drainage of tears

The lacrimal puncti (upper and lower) are at the medial canthus (see above) on the mucosal side of the eyelid margins and carry the tears through the upper and lower canaliculi, which join to form the nasolacrimal sac which leads into the nasolacrimal duct. This duct drains into the back of the throat, which explains why tears or eye-drops are 'tasted' at the back of the throat. Make sure that you memorise the diagram of the lacrimal apparatus (Fig. 2.4). It is very important to know this anatomy and vocabulary if, for example, you are going to learn how to do a lacrimal sac washout or assess an eyelid injury.

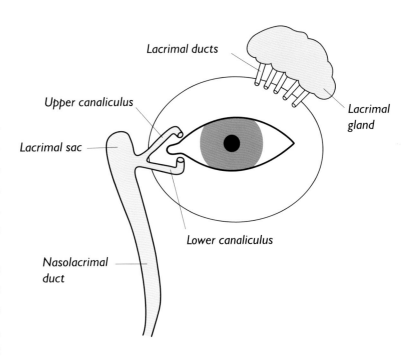

Figure 2.4 *The lacrimal apparatus.*

The conjunctiva

The conjunctiva is a transparent mucous membrane that lines the inner surfaces of the eyelids and folds back to cover the front surface of the eyeball, with the exception of the cornea. It contains tiny blood vessels that are visible to the naked eye. Its goblet cells secrete mucin, the inner layer of the tear film, which helps retain the middle, watery layer of the tears on the front of the eye.

You can see from Fig. 2.5 that the conjunctiva consists of three areas; it is important for you to remember the names of these in order to accurately describe and document the condition of a person's conjunctiva. First is the palpaebral conjunctiva. This is a moderately thick layer, attached to the inside of the eyelids. If it is healthy, it provides a smooth, moist, slippery surface to facilitate the movement of the eye within the socket. The upper and lower fornices where the conjunctiva folds back on itself are often described as 'pocket' like (Fig. 2.5). They fulfil the useful safety function of ensuring that dust, dirt and larger foreign bodies do not normally become lodged behind the eye. The superior fornices also contain the minor accessory glands of Krause and Wolfring that contribute to the tear film. The conjunctiva is relatively loose and folded in this area to facilitate free

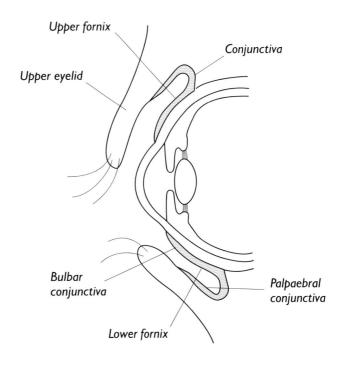

Figure 2.5 *The conjunctival fornices.*

movement of the eye and eyelids. The bulbar conjunctiva covers the anterior surface of the eye. It is relatively thin and translucent and is fairly loosely attached to the surface of the eye.

The limbus

At the limbus the conjunctiva is closely attached to the sclera (Fig. 2.1). It progressively transmutes until it is continuous with the cornea when it becomes the transparent epithelial outer layer of the cornea. Beneath the surface of the limbus lie the canal of Schlemm and the trabecular meshwork that communicates with channels called the 'aqueous veins' (they contain no blood, only aqueous), which in turn connect with the conjunctival veins in the area of the limbus (and drain aqueous into the venous system).

The sclera

This is the tough, outer white of the eye formed from fibrous tissue, elastic fibres and connective tissue. It is in continuity with the dura of the central nervous system. The sclera joins with the cornea at the limbus, and extends to the optic nerve at the back of the eye, where it is continuous with the dura. The external muscles of the eye are attached to the sclera, and its anterior surface is loosely covered by the conjunctiva.

The cornea

The cornea (Fig. 2.6) is composed of five layers:

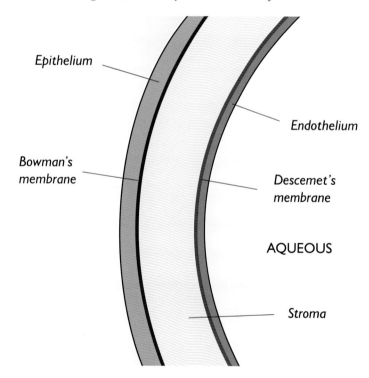

Figure 2.6 *The cornea.*

Epithelium: This is the thin outer surface of the cornea, and is only five or six cells thick. These cells contain no keratin so they must be kept moist all the time, or they will die. Corneal epithelial cells are naturally shed continuously into the tear film and are continuously replaced. In the event of an injury to the epithelium, this natural process is speeded up and an epithelial defect, depending on its size and location on the cornea, can heal rapidly with no scarring. The naked ends of unmyelinated nerve fibres run between the epithelial cells, making the corneal epithelium highly sensitive to pain.

Bowman's membrane: This lies under the epithelium, and consists of collagen fibres. This layer is relatively tough so it provides a little protection against deeper injuries. If the cornea is damaged at this layer, or deeper, a white scar will develop on healing.

Stroma: Stroma is the thickest layer, representing nearly 90% of the thickness of the cornea. It consists of many layers of collagen fibres arranged parallel to each other within each layer, and at right angles to the layers above and below. The special arrangement of the collagen fibres is one of the mechanisms for keeping the cornea transparent.

Descemet's membrane: This tough elastic membrane lies between the stroma and endothelium.

Corneal endothelium: This consists of a single layer of specialised cells that control hydration of the cornea in two ways, by limiting the amounts of aqueous passing into the stroma, and by actively pumping excess fluid from the stroma back into the aqueous. If these cells are damaged or diseased, they never regenerate.

To do ...

What are the cornea's two main functions?

The corneal **endothelium** has two very significant functions: it controls the movement of fluids and solutes through the cornea and it pumps excessive fluid out of the cornea to maintain its clarity. Ask a theatre nurse why viscoelastic preparations like Healon™, Amvisc™ and Rayvisc™ are used in relation to the corneal endothelium during intraocular surgery (if you cannot find anyone to help you, check Shunsuke *et al.*, 2005).

The normal cornea has no blood vessels, so what two means are responsible for supplying the cornea with oxygen, nutrition, and carrying away waste products?

The uveal tract

This is the collective term for the choroid, ciliary body and iris. You may hear patients referred to as having anterior or posterior uveitis.

The iris

When speaking to patients, the iris is often referred to as 'the coloured part' of the eye. It separates the anterior chamber from the posterior chamber) (Fig. 2.1). The colour of the iris is determined by the amount of melanin on the anterior face of the iris. If a lot of melanin is present, the iris will appear very dark brown, but if there is very little then it will look blue. The texture, colour and individual markings on the iris vary in form and character from one person to another and iris scans can be used as a unique means of identification for security purposes.

There are two groups of plain muscle fibres in the iris. The *sphincter pupillae* is, as its name suggests, a circular band of muscle that contracts and relaxes to vary the amount of light entering the eye. The *dilator pupillae* consists of strands of muscle fibres arranged like the spokes of a wheel, which contract to pull the iris open. Make a note of the full names of these two muscles as you must know them for the test at the end of this chapter. You must also understand what they do and how they work in order to grasp the basic pharmacology involved in dilating the pupil, and to know why particular eye-drops may be contraindicated for some people.

Stimulation of the sympathetic nervous system by events (e.g. fear or a sudden shock) or by drugs will cause the fibres of the dilator pupillae muscle to contract and cause dilatation of the pupils. Similarly, the parasympathetic system can be activated (e.g. by drugs or light stimulation) to cause constriction of the pupils.

Psychology and the pupil

Did you know that pupil size is an indication of sexual attraction, pain, surprise and fear (Bradley et al., 2008)? It can also indicate if someone has been using a controlled substance. As a health professional should you be looking at people's faces – and particularly their eyes – a little more closely?

The ciliary body

This structure is situated just behind the iris. Its pleated anterior surface – the *pars plicata* – is covered with ciliary processes that produce (through a filtration process) the *aqueous humour*, which is the clear fluid filling the anterior part of the eye. The aqueous humour is similar in composition to blood plasma and supplies nutrients and oxygen to the lens and cornea, which are both without a blood supply. Production and drainage of the aqueous fluid are normally balanced to maintain the *intraocular pressure* within the anterior chamber at between 10 and 21 mmHg in the average person. Intraocular pressure usually shows a diurnal variation of 2–3 mmHg, with the highest reading being in the early morning. The ciliary body also provides the anchor points for tiny fibres that are as delicate as gossamer, the *lens zonules*, which suspend the lens. The *pars plana* of the ciliary body contains the circular ciliary muscle. When this contracts and relaxes, the lens becomes thicker and thinner to focus the lens for near or distant vision.

To do ...

How does acetazolamide (Diamox™) work to reduce the production of aqueous? Check the NetDoctor and Patient UK websites.

The choroid

This is the vascular layer of the eye that lies between the retina and the sclera.

The lens

The cells of the lens are encased in a thick elastic capsule. The front part of the lens capsule, which sits behind the iris, is called the *anterior lens capsule*. The back part, which holds the vitreous in place, is called the *posterior lens capsule*. The lens is unusual in that it continues to produce new cells throughout life and because its original embryonic cells are not shed or absorbed, it grows slowly with age, and the centre of the lens, the lens nucleus, becomes harder and more compacted. In order to function well the lens needs to be both 'elastic' and transparent. The earliest ageing change is presbyopia, which affects the elasticity of the lens. Cataracts are common in older people.

To do ...

Write two sentences on presbyopia and how it is caused.
(Medline Plus and the Eye Digest website on the ageing eye will help you with this.)

To do ...

Consider the effect of a cycloplegic eye-drop on the focusing power of the lens (see Chapter 4 Basic Pharmacology). How would you advise a patient who has had a cycloplegic drop instilled?

The drainage angle

There are two means by which aqueous humour drains from the eye. You will see from Fig.2.7 that the aqueous humour fills the tiny posterior chamber behind the iris, flows through the pupil into the anterior chamber of the eye and is drained through the trabecular meshwork, into the canal of Schlemm and is collected by the conjunctival veins. This is known as the conventional drainage route, and by this means, 85–90% of the aqueous leaves the eye (Ahmed, 2004). This outflow system is responsible for regulating the intraocular pressure, as the mechanism is pressure sensitive.

Ahmed (2004) states that the uveoscleral drainage route is responsible for draining an estimated 5–15% of the aqueous via the stroma and vessels of the iris root and ciliary body, regardless of the intraocular pressure. Through the combination of the conventional route and the uveoscleral route, about 1% of the aqueous drains away per minute. It is important to have some understanding of these two drainage routes in order to understand the principles behind medical treatments for intraocular pressure.

The trabecular meshwork is also responsible for removing cellular debris from the anterior chamber by phagocytosis and is able to facilitate the removal of some debris into the canal of Schlemm (Buller *et al.*, 1990). It is thus generally able to clear red blood cells (hyphaema) and inflammatory products like hypopyon (pus in the anterior chamber).

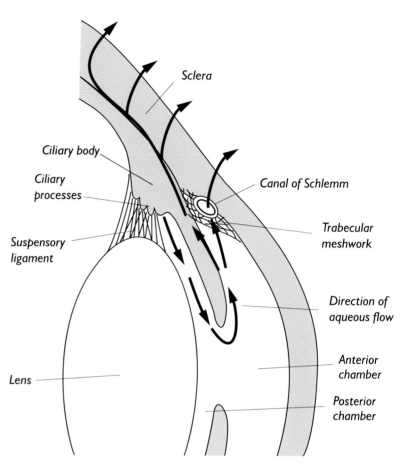

Figure 2.7 *Aqueous drainage.*

Vitreous humour

The vitreous occupies the space at the back of the eye, between the lens and the retina. It is a transparent gel-like substance that maintains the shape of the eye and holds the neural and pigment layers of the retina in position. It is composed of around 98% water and contains a network of collagen fibrils that maintain its shape. Unlike the aqueous, the vitreous is not continually produced and drained.

The retina

Critical to an understanding of retinal detachment is the fact that embryonic eyes develop from two optic vesicles which are derived from the embryonic forebrain. The retina and optic nerve develop from the optic cup, which folds in on itself; its outer wall develops into the retinal pigment epithelium, and the inner wall becomes the sensory layer of the retina. The retina therefore originally comprised two layers – the nervous layer and the pigment layer. Because of the nature of its embryonic development, the retina is thus an outward extension of the brain, to which it remains connected via the optic nerve (see Snell and Lemp, 1998).

The layers of the retina

The anterior surface of the *neural layer of the retina* is a thin, transparent sensory layer that lies in contact with the vitreous humour. It contains two types of photoreceptors – rods and cones. The *pigment layer* is a single layer of cells, which absorbs the light energy entering the eye. It delivers nutrition to the photoreceptors in the neural layer and has a key role in the chemical activity of the neural layer, which includes digesting, and recycling specialised cell products from the neural layer. It secretes a range of growth factors to maintain the visual function of the retina (Strauss, 2004).

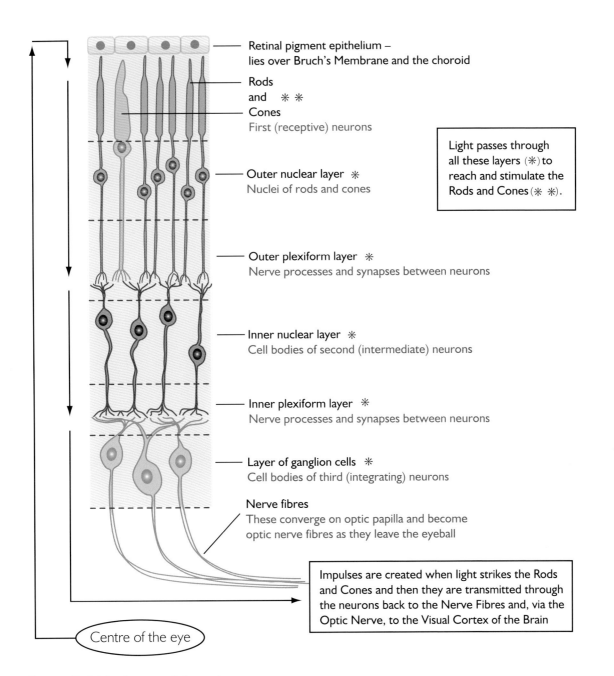

Figure 2.8 *The layers of the retina*

Key learning for the beginner

The **fundus** is the term used by ophthalmologists to describe the posterior part of the eyeball. It can be examined with an ophthalmoscope or a slit lamp using additional hand-held lenses. Within the fundal area are:

● the **optic disc**, where the **optic nerve**, the **central retinal artery** and the **central retinal vein** enter and leave the eye

● the **macula**, which is situated in the posterior part of the retina of each eye, and looks a slightly darker red than the surrounding retina. It is responsible for the clearest and most detailed colour vision.

In retinal detachment the neural layer of the retina peels away from the pigment layer. As you will already have noted from the above discussion, the retina developed as two distinct layers.

To do ...

Find out why people with retinal detachments are sometimes asked to maintain their heads in specific positions pre- and postoperatively.

Why do some retinal patients require treatment more urgently than others?

What are the functions of a) rods and b) cones?

The optic pathways

Many patients tend to think that we 'see' with our eyes, so all disturbances with our vision must necessarily fall within the remit of the ophthalmic department. This is not necessarily so. Consider briefly the development of the embryo, already discussed under the heading 'retina'. The eyes begin to develop 22 days after conception, with the formation of optic grooves in the early brain tissue, from which eventually two 'buds' (optic vesicles) may be seen on either side of the forebrain. Eventually these vesicles expand laterally, making stalk-like connections with the developing nervous system. These 'stalks' eventually become the optic nerves.

The optic nerves

Like the brain, the optic nerves are covered with the pia, arachnoid and dura maters. As you can see in Fig. 2.10, the optic nerves partially cross over at the optic chiasma. This partial separation of the nerve fibres from each eye allows the left side of the brain to interpret the left visual field, and the right side of the brain to interpret the right visual field. This enables the slightly different information coming from each eye to be interpreted together, to facilitate depth perception, and results in the highly complex process that psychologists call *visual perception*. This involves not just 'seeing' but also being able to make sense of what has been perceived.

Any lesion occurring in one or both optic nerves as they leave the eye will cause a loss of vision. The optic chiasma lies just above the pituitary gland, so any enlargement of this gland will put pressure on the crossed fibres, causing a bilateral temporal loss of vision (bitemporal hemianopia). You can find out more about loss of vision due to damage to the optic pathways in Miller *et al.* (2007).

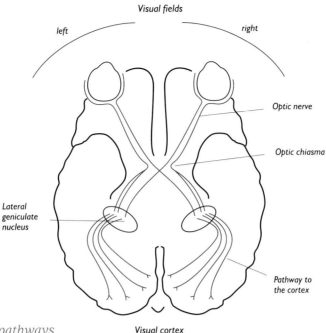

Figure 2.9 *The optic pathways.*

To do ...

Give three possible causes of partial loss of vision occurring as a result of optic nerve damage at the chiasma or following the separation of the nerve fibres as they proceed to the visual cortex of the brain.

Loss of vision occurring as a result of damage to the optic pathways is not generally an ophthalmic problem, but patients who complain primarily of a loss of vision are generally seen in the ophthalmic department where the health of the retina may be ascertained and the visual fields recorded for diagnostic purposes. Many ophthalmic departments run joint ophthalmic neurological clinics.

References and further reading

Ahmed, E. (2004). *A Textbook of Ophthalmology.* India: Prentice-Hall.

Bradley, M., Miccoli, L., Escrig, M. and Lang, P. (2008). The pupil as a measure of emotional arousal and autonomic activation. *Psychophysiology*, 45(4), 602–07.

BMJ Publishing Group and Royal Pharmaceutical Society of Great Britain (2008). *British National Formulary.* Biggleswade, UK: RPS Publishing.

Buller, C., Johnson, D. and Tschumper, R. (1990). Human trabecular meshwork phagocytosis. *Investigative Ophthalmology and Visual Science*, 31(10), 2156–63.

Marsden, J. (2008). *An Evidence Base for Ophthalmic Practice.* Chichester: John Wiley.

Miller, N., Newman, N., Biousse, V. and Kerrison, J. (2007). *Walsh and Hoyt's Clinical Neuro-Ophthalmology: The Essentials*, 2nd edn. London: Wolters Kluwer Health.

Moore, J., Graham, J., Goodall, E., *et al.* (2009). Concordance between common dry eye diagnostic tests. *British Journal of Ophthalmology*, 93(1), 66–72.

Shunsuke, T., Shen'Ichiro, Y., Chrisato, M., *et al.* (2005). Protective effect on the corneal epithelium and remaining efficiency at the anterior chamber for three different kinds of viscoelastic devices. *Japanese Journal of Ophthalmic Surgery*, 18(3), 409–12.

Snell, R. and Lemp, M. (1998). *Clinical Anatomy of the Eye*, 2nd edn. Oxford: Blackwell Science.

Strauss, O. (2004). The retinal pigment epithelium in visual function. *Physiological Reviews*, 85(3), 845–81.

Useful web resources

Ageing Eye.net

http://www.ageingeye.net

See the Eye Digest for more detailed information about the ageing eye.

BBC Health: Ask the Doctor

http://www.bbc.co.uk/health/ask_the_doctor/

National Library of Medicine (US) Medline Plus

http://medlineplus.gov

For information on presbyopia.

NetDoctor UK

http://www2.netdoctor.co.uk

For information on acetazolamide.

Patient UK

http://www.patient.co.uk

For information on dry eyes and carbonic anhydrase inhibitors.

VetMed Resource

http://www.cababstractsplus.org/veterinarymedicine/

Article by T. Caceci on the anatomy and physiology of the eye and development of the eye in invertebrates.

SELF TEST *answers on page 203*

1. Label this diagram of the eye.

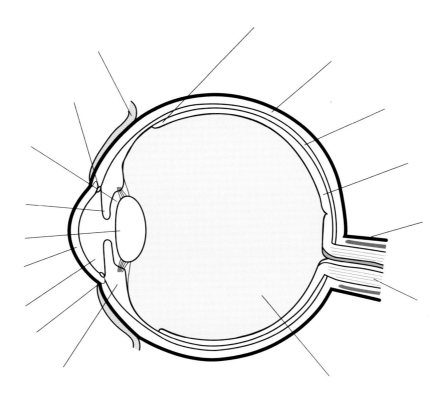

2. What are the tiny openings in the corners of the eyelids called?

_____

3. Where are the reflex tears produced?

_____

4. What is the function of mucin, produced by the goblet cells of the conjunctiva?

_____

_____

5. The conjunctival glands of Krause and Wolfring, situated in the upper and lower fornices, are responsible for secreting what?

_____

_____

6. The cornea is composed of five layers. What is the inner, endothelial layer responsible for?

7. What is the uveal tract composed of?

8. Name the two muscles of the iris.

9. What are the main functions of the ciliary body?

10. What is presbyopia?

11. What anatomical structures are involved in the 'conventional' drainage route from the eye?

12. What is the name of the other route for the drainage of aqueous from the eye?

13. Name the two main layers of the retina

14. What four key structures are at 'the fundus'?

_____

_____

15. What are the cones in the retina responsible for?

_____

_____

16. The fibres from the optic nerve cross over at an area lying just above the pituitary gland. What is this called?

_____

Chapter 3

Basic refraction

Dorothy Field

Sight is our most important sense. Without sight, we would be unlikely to survive without help. The *quality* of a person's vision significantly affects the way they manage their daily life, as many common tasks like cooking are more difficult if, for example, the long-sighted cook has no reading glasses; similarly a customer in a restaurant cannot read a menu without reading glasses. Understanding how light is refracted within the eye is key to understanding the visual needs of our patients, particularly when it comes to obtaining accurate intraocular lens readings and understanding spectacle prescriptions and associated visual difficulties.

Essential learning

If you normally work with cataract patients, it is essential that you begin to get a grasp of the following:

● The vocabulary common when discussing refraction.

● How the eye works to focus images on the retina.

● Some of the pitfalls associated with inaccurate measurements prior to cataract surgery, or the insertion of a lens of the incorrect power (see Chapters 5, 6 and 7).

What is refraction?

Refraction of light by the eye to produce good, unaided vision (by focusing the light on to the retina) is dependent on the power of the cornea, the lens and the length of the eye. All the individual transparent areas of the eye contribute to bending and focusing the light rays on the retina. Snell and Lemp (1998) state that the power of the whole normal (emmetropic) eye is about 58 dioptres (see Dioptre in Appendix 2); the cornea has a refractive power of about 42 dioptres and is responsible for more than two-thirds of this refractive ability. In addition it should be recognised that the tear film, aqueous humour, lens and vitreous all contribute to refraction of the light rays so that they normally come to a focus at the macula.

The lens only contributes about 15 dioptres to the total refractive power of the eye. The significance of the lens is that it can change its dioptric power by contraction and relaxation of the ciliary muscle. This is because the lens becomes thicker (more convex) when the ciliary muscle contracts and thinner when it relaxes. Contraction of the ciliary muscle releases the tension on the zonule fibres, allowing the lens to increase its curvature. This process of changing the lens shape is called accommodation, and it allows distant and near objects to be focused on the retina. The amount by which the lens can change in power reduces with age – about 8 dioptres at the age of 40 and only 1–2 dioptres at the age of 60 (Snell and Lemp, 1998).

Focusing the eye for near vision

This involves:

Pupil constriction: Smaller pupil diameters result in an increased depth of focus and an improved retinal image.

Convergence: This is when the eyes turn slightly inwards towards the nose, and it ensures that the image is projected on to the fovea of each eye, aiding binocular vision and increasing 3-D perception (stereopsis).

Accommodation: When we look at objects near to us, *diverging* light rays reach our corneas so the eye requires more refractive power to focus the light on to the retina (but parallel light rays come from objects in the distance). This is illustrated in Fig. 3.1.

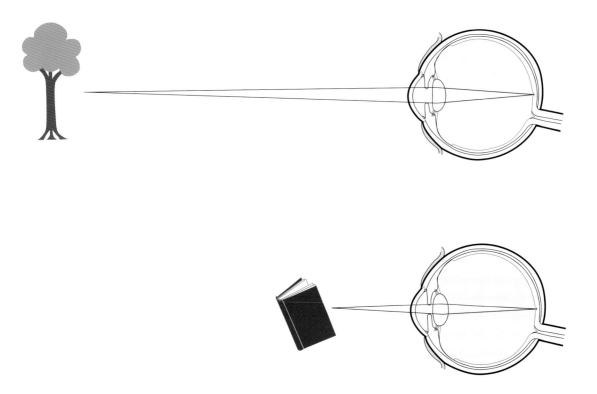

Figure 3.1 *Viewing a distant object (top) and viewing a near object (below)*

To focus on a near object the lens needs to become thicker (i.e. have a greater dioptric power and a shorter focal length). In order to do this, the ciliary muscles contract, making a smaller ring, and taking the tension off the suspensory ligaments. This means the lens becomes smaller and fatter and moves slightly backwards, to increase refraction. The ciliary muscles are innervated by the autonomic nervous system, and accommodation is controlled automatically by the brain.

When the lens needs to become thinner for distance vision, the ciliary body relaxes, pulling the zonule fibres taut, so the lens is under tension and becomes flatter and returns to its slightly forward position.

You can read more about the process of accommodation at the websites of Georgia State University HyperPhysics and *Ted Montgomery*.

Emmetropia (normal sight)

The refractive components of the normal eye are able to focus light from a distant object (parallel light) on the retina accurately, so that the person is able to see distant objects clearly without spectacles. When a person is young and has 'normal' accommodation they will also be able to read without spectacles. However, with age even 'normal'-sighted people have decreased ability to accommodate (presbyopia) which means that spectacles will be needed for close work.

Ammetropia (refractive error)

This term indicates a variation in the shape of the eye that interferes with accurate light refraction. Refractive errors generally occur as a result of eye shape rather than disease. Factors affecting the possibility of someone having (or developing) a refractive error include their age, whether their parents were long- or short-sighted, their race and the environment they live and work in. For example, people who live and work for days in confined spaces such as underwater diving bells and submarines tend to develop myopia (see below). This may pass off to some extent following a return to a normal environment (Onoo *et al.*, 2002).

Myopia (short-sightedness)

A myopic eye (Fig. 3.2) may have an eyeball that is longer than normal or have a cornea that is too convex so that the light rays come to a focus in front of the retina. The result is that close objects look clear, while objects further away look blurred.

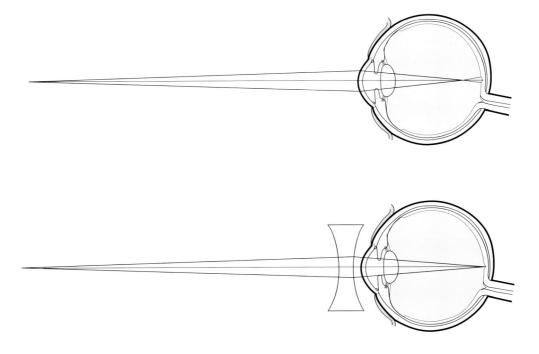

Figure 3.2 *Uncorrected myopia (top) and corrected myopia (below).*

To do ...

Myopia is increasing in modern social environments.

· Visit the NHS National Library for Health and use the search term 'myopia increasing modern society' to try to discover some of the factors influencing this change. Check out the article by Saw *et al.* (1996) to find out whether myopia might be linked to intelligence, demographic patterns or genetic factors.

Why do you think many ophthalmologists have a tendency to short-sightedness? Are there any advantages to this?

Hypermetropia (long-sightedness)

A hypermetropic eyeball (Fig. 3.3) may be shorter than normal or the cornea may not be convex enough. When looking into the distance the person must use the natural power of their lens to see clearly. Because the hypermetropic person already has to use most of their natural focusing power to see in the distance, they are less able to see near objects clearly.

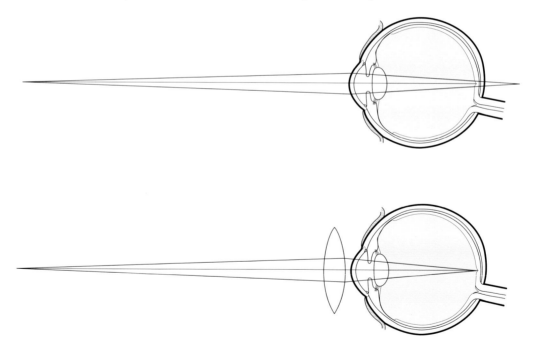

Figure 3.3 *Uncorrected hypermetropia (top) and corrected hypermetropia (below).*

As with short sight, long sight is usually inherited. Babies and young children tend to be naturally slightly long-sighted. As they grow, the eye lengthens a little and their hypermetropia reduces. As young people they can often use the focusing power of their eyes to overcome the problem of hypermetropia. However, in their late teens and early 20s, the lens begins to become a little harder and they may then require spectacles. If you have hypermetropia, your prescription will have a positive value (for example, +2.25 dioptres).

Astigmatism

Astigmatism (Fig. 3.4) is caused when the front of the eye is not completely spherical. It can be because the cornea or lens curves more in one direction than in the other, with resulting distortion when viewing both distant and near objects. It is possible to have some degree of astigmatism in one or both eyes, as well as being either hypermetropic or myopic. It is a fairly stable condition, which changes only slightly over a lifetime. Any eye surgery that involves a corneal incision can create or alter astigmatism.

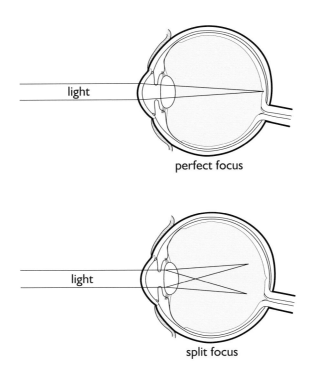

Figure 3.4 *Corrected astigmatism (top) and uncorrected astigmatism (below).*

Anisometropia

This is normally a congenital condition in which the two eyes have unequal refractive powers. A person might be very hypermetropic in one eye, and less so in the other. One eye may even be myopic and the other hypermetropic.

Anisometropia in a young child can cause amblyopia (in anisometropia the amblyopia normally only affects one eye). Amblyopia develops because eyes can only accommodate by an equal amount. If the eyes have unequal refractive powers one eye will normally receive a clearer image than the other. For example if a child's right eye is + 1.00 and his or her left eye is + 3.00, then both eyes will accommodate by + 1.00 dioptre. The right eye will then be focused but the image in the left eye will remain 2 dioptres out of focus. The brain will concentrate on using the vision from the eye with a more focused image (in this example the right eye), but will not use the less focused image from the other eye as much (in this example the left eye). The eye with the less focused image becomes amblyopic (or *lazy*) because vital visual connections in the brain are not stimulated to form images. Amblyopia develops in childhood as the brain's visual connections mature with age. By the age of about 8 years the potential for good vision will remain even if anisometropia develops, but any amblyopia already present will remain throughout life. Different image sizes are of course, only one of several reasons for the development of amblyopia in children.

In adults, a difference in the required spectacle prescription of both eyes of about 3 dioptres can lead to diplopia (double vision) as the brain will perceive a different sized image from each eye and there will be different optical effects in each eye from the unequal spectacle lenses that the brain finds difficult to interpret. The brain is unable to fuse these images into a single picture, and the patient may be very uncomfortable, possibly needing to cover one eye to walk around safely. This may occur intentionally if a surgeon deliberately corrects a significant refractive error in a patient's first eye during cataract surgery, knowing that the second eye needs to be operated on soon after. For example a person who is –6.00 preoperatively in both eyes may become –1.00 (or even 'normal') for distance vision in their postoperative eye. When this is done, the patient will need surgery on their second eye promptly to 're-balance' the eyes. Normally the surgeon and clinic nurse will discuss these problems with the patient preoperatively. If the person has only one cataract, the ophthalmologist will generally ensure that the postoperative refraction matches the unoperated eye as closely as possible.

Accurate preoperative measurements for lens implants are essential. A wrong lens prescription can cause a patient to have an unexpected refractive problem. Similarly, very careful checking of the lens implant at the time of surgery is vital, as any mistake with biometry procedures or the insertion of a lens of the wrong power could result in a requirement for further surgery, or even litigation.

Presbyopia (ageing eyes)

The lens of the eye continues to grow throughout life, and its inner fibres become tightly compacted. The lens becomes less flexible and therefore its shape is less able to be changed via contraction and relaxation of the ciliary muscle. These changes start to become noticeable by the time a person reaches their 40s. Because the lens no longer focuses for near vision as well as it used to, the person will begin to hold their reading material (e.g. the daily newspaper) further away from their face in an attempt to read. Eventually reading spectacles or bifocal lenses will be needed. On average, the strength of reading spectacles required to correct presbyopia is +1.5 to +2.50 dioptres. Check this out next time you see a display of reading spectacles in a shop.

Correction of refractive errors

Spectacles are the cheapest means of dealing with a refractive problem, causing no harm to the eye. Plastic lenses may also offer a degree of protection in an accident situation. Contact lenses carry regular expense and a number of risk factors. LASIK (laser in situ keratomileusis) is a means of changing the shape of the cornea to compensate for a refractive problem. It is becoming increasingly popular.

There are many reasons why people choose to wear contact lenses. These include the freedom to participate more fully in sports, their personal appearance and peer pressure. However, people with a high degree of myopia or considerable hypermetropia wish to see more clearly without the often troublesome optical effects of high-powered spectacle lenses. People with very high prescriptions are only able to have clear vision through the centre of their spectacle lenses, and these lenses are often unattractive and restrict the choice of spectacle frames.

Objective and subjective refraction

There are various ways of testing a patient's eyes for spectacles.

Objective refraction

Objective refraction does not need any response from the patient and is obtained from:

- Cycloplegic refraction: This may be used for young children and babies as well as people with learning difficulties. Cyclopentolate eye-drops are instilled to prevent accommodation (an additional effect of these drops is to dilate the pupil). The patient is then examined with a retinoscope (see below). Babies and young children may be refracted while anaesthetised (if anaesthetised for other reasons). This is why theatre staff may need a lens box when a child is being examined under anaesthetic.

- Retinoscopy: An optometrist or ophthalmologist uses a retinoscope to observe the direction of reflected light from the retina. Neutralising the light movement using trial lenses gives an indication of the power of the eye. Adults are asked to relax their eyes in a darkened room and look at a green light at the end of the room. This stops them changing the focus of their eyes during the examination. For an experienced professional this is a quick and accurate method for generating a prescription. People who have had cyclopentolate eye-drops are asked to look straight at the retinoscope light because they are unable to accommodate.

See Chua's Eye Page to understand what the optometrist is looking for during retinoscopy.

Subjective refraction

This is when the optometrist asks a patient to respond to changes in the power of lenses, by asking if vision is clearer or more blurred with, for example, lens one or lens two. It is normal for an optometrist to examine both objectively and subjectively. They are checking that the prescription is accurate in order to provide the patient with clear comfortable vision.

Generating an optical prescription

Many people in our society wear spectacles or contact lenses to achieve clear vision. A short explanation follows of how an optical prescription is generated. The basic equipment required includes a lens box, a trial frame and a retinoscope.

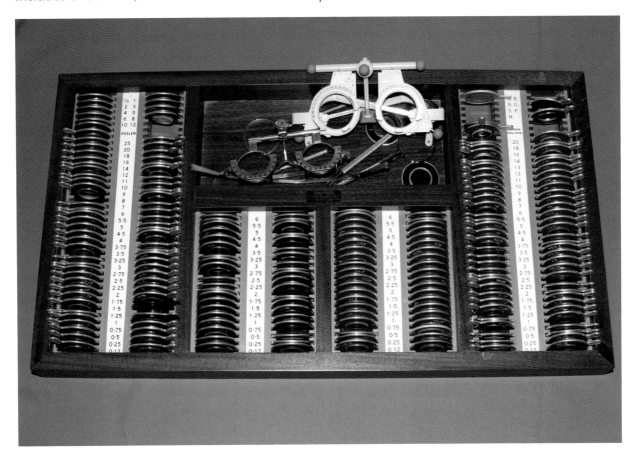

Figure 3.5 *Lens box and trial frame*
© Samantha Hartley, Ophthalmic Photographer, Royal Bournemouth Hospital, UK.

The **trial frame** is an adjustable spectacle frame constructed to accommodate the trial lenses that the optometrist uses during the examination. It is adjusted to suit the patient's head size and facial features so that they will be looking through the centre of the lenses used throughout the test.

The **phoropter** is a complex piece of apparatus that can be used instead of a trial frame and a box of individual lenses. It is more usual to see this in use in an optometrist's clinic than in a hospital eye department.

The **dioptre** is an internationally standardised unit used by optometrists and ophthalmologists for prescribing lenses, using the metric system. One dioptre (+ or –) will adjust a person's focusing distance by 1 metre, so even a relatively low prescription can give positive patient benefits for driving and reading. A simple plus or minus lens is known as a *sphere*. The power of the lenses prescribed can be measured in quarter dioptre stages to two decimal places (e.g. + 2.25 or –3.75). Most average myopic (short-sighted) people have spectacle lenses of –2.00 to –3.00, and very myopic people (high myopes) may have lenses measuring –10.00. Hypermetropic (long-sighted) people will have plus (+) prescriptions of similar strengths. A standard table for recording optical prescriptions is shown in Table 3.1.

Table 3.1 *Optical prescriptions.*

	Sphere	Cyl.	Axis	Prism	Base	Add
R.						
L.						

The **cylinder** (you may also hear this referred to as a *cyl*) is a lens used to correct astigmatism. If you have an astigmatism, the dioptric power of the lens will be noted in the cylinder box of the prescription form (see above). The greater the astigmatic correction, the greater the difference between the two focusing planes of the eye. The cylinder is a specialised lens which focuses light in one direction only; turning the lens round on its axis (central line) will change the direction in which it focuses. The *axis number* indicates the number of degrees from the horizontal position (0–180°) that the cylinder lens has to be rotated within the trial frame to produce clear vision for the patient.

The Jackson crossed-cylinder technique is normally used to check the correct axis (position) and consists of a lens divided into two, with one meridian being a negative power and the other meridian being a positive power. Turning the lens over will cause a change in the quality of the image the patient perceives between the two meridians if the cylinder is not in the correct position.

A **prism** is used to direct the rays of light without altering their focus, and is used to increase convergence when prescribing reading spectacles or bifocal reading prescriptions. Prisms are also used to re-align the light rays for people with mild squints.

The **base** information on a prescription indicates the direction of the prism and it gives a reference point regarding which direction the image is being moved in (recorded as up or down or in or out).

The **reading additions** are used on top of the general prescription to improve the near vision of people with presbyopia, normally between + 1.50 and + 2.50. When the spectacles are made up, the reading addition is added to the power of the distance lens.

In addition to objective and subjective refraction as a means of arriving at a spectacle prescription, an *autorefractor* may be used in a hospital clinic setting to provide an almost instant objective refraction, for the purposes of:

- Diagnosis (e.g. poor vision following cataract surgery which may be as a result of a large post-operative astigmatism).

- Approximate prescription (a patient may have forgotten to bring their spectacles and appropriate corrective lenses are often required to enable accurate testing of visual fields). Using the information from the autorefractor, trial lenses can be used instead of spectacles for the test.

It is not envisaged that an autorefractor will ever replace the function of the optometrist, as careful objective and subjective refraction is the most reliable means of generating a spectacle prescription, particularly when a cylinder is being used to correct astigmatism.

Types of spectacles

Single-vision lenses

These are prescribed for younger people who are either short-sighted (myopic) or long-sighted (hypermetropic) for all their daily activities. They still have enough flexibility in the natural lens of their eyes to accommodate (focus) for near vision requirements. Short-sighted people may have such good near vision that they take their spectacles off to view very tiny objects. Single-vision lenses are considered to be relatively inexpensive.

Bifocal lenses

These spectacle lenses are used to correct presbyopia for people who have been spectacle wearers for most of their lives (see above). They have a prescription lens for distance vision at the top, and a lens with a different prescription at the bottom. These spectacles are recognisable by a line that runs all or part of the way across the lens. They are more expensive than single-vision lenses, but are more convenient and probably cheaper than buying two pairs of spectacles.

Varifocal lenses

These gradually change focus and do not have a hard line between the distance and reading sections. Because they merge two lens prescriptions gradually, they are capable of producing clearer mid-range vision, depending on the position of the person's eye behind the lens. To be most effective, the lenses need to be reasonably large and require to be expertly fitted within the spectacle frame. Depending on their normal activities, people will be either delighted with their vision or dissatisfied with the size of the reading or distance area of the lens.

Ready-readers

Patients who do not need correction for seeing at a distance can receive a prescription for reading glasses or buy them over the counter to correct presbyopia. It is important that people who buy so-called ready-readers also know to make an appointment with the optometrist for full eye examinations so that the health of their eyes can be checked every couple of years.

Unfortunately many people use ready-readers for years without seeing an optometrist for a health check of their eyes, where problems such as glaucoma can be detected. Given that some of these eye problems damage eyesight irrecoverably if untreated, health professionals should recommend regular 2-yearly eye examinations to all people over the age of 40.

To do …

Check out your own spectacle prescription (if you wear them) on the departmental focimeter.

Practise feeling your patients' spectacles to see if they are minus (concave in shape) or plus (convex in shape). Remember to polish them afterwards! This can be a useful observation to make as some eye problems are linked to long- or short-sightedness.

Ask your mentor or departmental optometrist to show you the different lenses that are used for eye tests.

Make sure that you can distinguish between distance spectacles, reading spectacles, bifocals and varifocals. This is particularly important when you are testing a patient's vision.

Conclusions

Not only is it important that you understand the basics of refraction to understand variable spectacle prescriptions, but you also need to remember that some eye conditions may be linked to refractive errors. For example, people who develop retinal detachments are more likely to be myopic, and those developing primary acute closed-angle glaucoma will tend to be long-sighted. It is very important to understand a little about refraction when using the IOLMaster™.

It is essential in cataract surgery to know the overall power of the eye and how the different components contribute to this overall power in order to choose the right intraocular lens implant. This is why K readings of corneal curvatures are measured in two meridians. It is vital to consider both eyes (see *Anisometropia* above) in order to identify possibly inaccurate readings (see Chapter 5).

References and further reading

Jacobi, F., Zrenner, E., Broqhammer, M. and Pusch C. (2005). A genetic perspective on myopia. *Cell and Molecular Life Science*, 62(7/8), 800–08.

Onoo, A., Kiyosawa, M., Takase, H. and Mano, Y. (2002). Development of myopia as a hazard for workers in pneumatic caissons. *British Journal of Ophthalmology*, 86, 1274–77.

Saw, S-M., Katz, J., Schein, O., Chew, S-J. and Chan, T-K. (1996). Epidemiology of myopia. *Epidemiological Reviews*, 18(2), 175–82.

Snell, R. and Lemp, M. (1998). *Clinical Anatomy of the Eye*. Oxford: Blackwell Science.

Useful web resources

Chua's Eye Page: Success in MRCOphth
http://www.mrcophth.com/chua1.html
For more on retinoscopy, look at the animated clips.

Georgia State University Hyperphysics
http://hyperphysics.phy-astr.gsu.edu/Hbase/hph.html
See more about accommodation in the section on light and vision.

NHS Evidence Health Information (formerly NHS National Library for Health)
http://www.library.nhs.uk/
This provides a vast range of evidence-based health information, government guidance and research papers for NHS employees.

Ted Montgomery
http://www.tedmontgomery.com/the_eye/
Interactive site covering anatomy, physiology and pathology of the human eye, with tests you can practice on.

OphthoBook
http://www.ophthobook.com/
A free online book with a free video of a retinoscopy, plus other useful information.

SELF TEST *answers on page 203*

1. What four transparent areas within the eyeball are responsible for refracting light within the eye?

2. Focusing the eyes requires three processes. What are they?

3. Emmetropia is another name for what?

4. What are the medical terms for long sight and short sight, respectively?

5. Sometimes the corneal curvature is slightly irregular. What is this called?

6. What is the medical term for double vision?

7. Is a mydriatic refraction an objective or subjective refraction?

8. What is the name given to a simple plus or minus lens?

9. What is a cylinder (cyl.) used to correct?

10. What word beginning with 'p' might be something that is used in spectacles to correct a mild squint?

11. What is a 'reading addition' used for?

Chapter 4
Basic pharmacology
Julie Tillotson and Dorothy Field

Drugs for the management of ophthalmic conditions are available in the form of eye-drops, ointment and oral preparations. Eye-drops and ointment are both absorbed into the systemic circulation and should therefore be given the same respect and consideration as any other drug. For this reason it is important that nurses new to ophthalmology should have a good working knowledge of all the drugs commonly used, as well as their effects, their side effects, contraindications and possible interactions with other drugs.

 Most hospital Trusts have access to an online version of the British National Formulary through the hospital's intranet and pharmacy department sites. Alternatively you can go to the British National Formulary Online and register for personal access. The Electronic Medicines Compendium is another useful website for accessing drug information, which gives a summary of product characteristics (SPC) and the patient information leaflet (PIL) for each drug.

Eye-drops – the potential dangers of systemic absorption

In 1994 a report by Urtti *et al.* reminded medical professionals that eye-drops might be absorbed systemically and in sufficient amounts to cause potentially hazardous effects. Cautions continue to be issued, particularly regarding the use of eye-drops in babies and children

 See the Neonatal Formulary 5 website.

The problem arises because many drugs (like phenylephrine) are absorbed directly into the bloodstream via the blood vessels of the conjunctiva and the mucosa of the nasolacrimal duct. Consider the example of glyceryl trinitrate medications, which are absorbed systemically via the mouth. Drugs that are given orally are often coated in order to delay absorption, and are extensively metabolised by the digestive tract and liver. Phenylephrine in the eye-drop formulation is particularly hazardous in very young babies and children and some older people because it is absorbed via the conjunctival blood vessels without prior mediation by the liver.

Allergies

Always remember to document *all* your patient's allergies because some eye ointments (e.g. chloramphenicol) have a lanolin (wool fat) base. Some people are quite allergic to this substance.

The **British National Formulary** does not state the carrier base for ophthalmic ointments, so you need to look in the patient information leaflets to be sure if it contains lanolin or not.

Do advise parents that eye-drops should not be used for more than 4 weeks after first opening because of the risk of inadvertent contamination of the contents. Most eye-drops, except minims, contain preservatives to inhibit the growth of micro-organisms within the bottle. Some eye lubricants are now available preservative-free in bottles with 3-month disposal dates. The preservatives used are generally either benzalkonium chloride or thiomersal, but unfortunately some patients develop allergies to them, particularly in patients with very dry eyes who have been using a lot of eye-drops over a long period of time. Preservatives are absorbed by soft contact lenses. The soft lenses may, as a result, become toxic to the eye after a period of time. Therefore contact-lens wearers should be advised to wear spectacles for the duration of their eye-drop treatment. People wearing 'bandage contact lenses' should be issued with preservative-free eye-drops.

Minim is a word used to describe a tiny container of preservative-free eye-drops intended for a single use. If, for example, a soft contact lens wearer required these drops for use at home, the hospital pharmacy would commonly issue one minim per day; therefore these drops must be stored carefully between uses in the refrigerator, and discarded at the end of the day.

SELF-LEARNING

The following 'self-learning' section involves you in researching your own answers to the questions posed. Use the British National Formulary online at work to get your basic information, and make some brief but relevant notes for yourself on the following questions. You can ask colleagues to help you with some of the more difficult ones, but do try to answer them all, even if it takes some time. When you have finished the work for this chapter, make it a habit to thoroughly check into each 'new' ophthalmic preparation you encounter professionally. As you mature in ophthalmic nursing practice, you might also check to see if your hospital library has a copy of Bartlett and Jaanus (2007).

To do ...

You may prefer to use your folder as well as, or instead of, this workbook for this section.

Phenylephrine eye-drops

- What strengths is phenylephrine available in? Why?

 2.5% or 10%.

- Is phenylephrine a mydriatic or a cycloplegic drug and what is the difference? How does it work, and on which iris muscle?

- What do you need to think about if asked to use phenylephrine in a child? Check your answers with a pharmacist, an ophthalmologist and an ophthalmic nurse to get a grip on this important issue.

● What are the cautions required regarding the use of phenylephrine in adults?

● On discharge, what advice would you give to adult patients about the side effects they may experience?

Cyclopentolate eye-drops

● Does cyclopentolate have another name?

● What strength is cyclopentolate available in, and why?

● Is it a mydriatic or a cycloplegic and what is the difference?

● How does it work, and on which iris muscle?

● Can it be used for babies and children?

- Are there any potential drug interactions?

- Does cyclopentolate have any side effects?

- What advice would you give to patients on the side effects?

Pilocarpine eye-drops

- What strengths is pilocarpine available in?

  2% or 4%

- What does a miotic drug do?

  Make the pupil ~~eye~~ smaller.

- How does it work, and on which iris muscle?

- Can it be used for babies and children?

- Are there any potential drug interactions?

  Yes - corticosteroids Antihistamines Pethidine

- Does pilocarpine have any side effects?   Tricyclic anti depressants
  Local
  Burning itching stinging blurring of vision
       Browaches or headache

- What is pilocarpine used for these days?

Latanoprost eye-drops

- Does latanoprost have another name?

- What eye problem is latanoprost used to treat?

- What group of drugs does latanoprost belong to?

- How does it reduce the intraocular pressure? Relate this knowledge to what you have learned about aqueous drainage in Chapter 2.

- Are there any potential drug interactions?

- Does latanoprost have any side effects?

- What advice would you give to a patient about the side effects?

Acetazolamide injection and tablets

- What is acetazolamide used for in ophthalmology?

- What is the other name for this drug?

- Which area of the eye does it act on?

- Does it have any side effects?

- How would you advise a patient on the side effects?

- Are there any potential drug interactions?

- What is the normal oral dose?

- What is the normal intravenous dose?

- What is the maximum dose of acetazolamide that can be given in 24 hours?

- Why is it unsuitable for long-term use?

- If used in the longer term, what must be monitored?

Iodipine eye-drops

- What is iodipine used for in ophthalmology?

- What is its other name?

- Which area of the eye does it act on?

- Are there any cautions regarding driving?

- How would you advise a patient on these?

- Are there any potential drug interactions?

Oxybuprocaine eye-drops

- Does oxybuprocaine have another name?

- What is oxybuprocaine used for?

- How long does it act for?

- How would you advise a patient whose eye has been instilled with oxybuprocaine?

Tetracaine eye-drops

- Does tetracaine have another name?

  Amethocaine hydrochloride

- What is it used for?

  numb the eye

- How long does it act for?

- How would you advise a patient when tetracaine has been used in their eye?

Timolol eye-drops

- Are timolol drops sometimes known by another name?

- What eye problem is timolol used to treat?

- What group of drugs does timolol belong to?

- How does it reduce the intraocular pressure?

- Are there any potential drug interactions?

- Does timolol have any side effects and how important is the person's health history?

- Why are people on timolol eye-drops advised to compress their tear ducts following administration?

- Which other ophthalmic products contain timolol?

Chloramphenicol eye-drops

- Does chloramphenicol have another name?

- What group of drugs does chloramphenicol belong to?

- What eye problems is chloramphenicol used to treat?

- Are there any cautions in the use of chloramphenicol? If so, what are these?

- Is chloramphenicol suitable for children?

- Can chloramphenicol be used for pregnant and nursing mothers?

Fluorescein eye-drops and intravenous injection

- What group of preparations does fluorescein belong to?

- Why is fluorescein used in ophthalmology?

- Are there any cautions in the use of fluorescein?

- Are fluorescein eye-drops suitable for children?

- Can fluorescein eye-drops be used for pregnant and nursing mothers?

- What are the major adverse reactions associated with intravenous fluorescein injections?

- Read your department's protocol for fluorescein angiography.

Providing and prescribing eye medication

Nursing staff have been expanding their role for many years within ophthalmology and provide medication for patients using Patient Group Directions (PGDs). In May 2006 the UK Government extended the prescribing rights of nursing staff to include any licensed medication for any medical condition (except controlled drugs), which has been extremely beneficial in ophthalmology (Marsden, 2007).

Concluding activities

Find out the general principles of Patient Group Directions (PGDs). What groups of patients are PGDs suitable for? Does your ophthalmic unit use PGDs? If so, what eye conditions and drugs are covered and which members of the nursing team use them?

Try looking at the British National Formulary Online under the section General Guidance, and the NHS Prescribing Centre Patient Group Directions.

To do ...

Find out if your ophthalmic unit has a Non-Medical Prescriber. What is his or her role? Consider how being a Non-Medical Prescriber would affect your accountability in terms of clinical and legal responsibility.

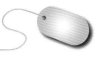

Go to the website for the National Prescribing Centre and look up Nurse Prescribing which gives the key principles and latest news on nurse prescribing.

References and further reading

Bartlett, J. and Jaanus, S. (2007). *Clinical Ocular Pharmacology*, 5th edn. Oxford: Butterworth Heineman.

Marsden, J. (2007). *An Evidence Base for Ophthalmic Nursing Practice*. Chichester: John Wiley.

Urtti, A., Rouhiainen, H., Kaila, T. and Saano, V. (1994). Controlled ocular timolol delivery. *Pharmaceutical Research*, 11(9), 1278–82.

Useful web resources

British National Formulary
http://www.bnf.org/bnf/

National Prescribing Centre
http://www.npc.co.uk/prescribers/index.htm

Neonatal Formulary 5
http://www.blackwellpublishing.com/medicine/bmj/nnf5/pdfs/comment/Eye_drops.pdf

NHS National Prescribing Centre: Patient Group Directions
www.npc.co.uk/publications/pgd/pgd.pdf
A practical guide and framework of competencies for all professionals using patient group directions (PGDs).

Patient Group Directions
http://www.portal.nelm.nhs.uk/PGD/default.aspx

Chapter 5

Preoperative cataract information

Claire Adams and Dorothy Field

This chapter offers considerable detail on the subject of cataracts, and is intended for those whose primary area of practice is within a preoperative ophthalmic clinic. It presents high-quality information around the preoperative cataract journey, that will help new staff provide patient-centred care within an efficient, cost-effective framework. It is also intended to be read as an overview by new ophthalmic theatre staff to understand why some patients are designated as 'consultant cases' and to anticipate potential intraoperative surgical difficulties.

A cataract is simply an opacity of the lens that produces alterations in visual perception. It is a painless and progressive condition which – if not treated – will result in gradual loss of useful vision. Perception of light will be maintained. Cataracts are the commonest potentially curable cause of blindness in the world.

Congenital cataracts

The Royal National Institute for the Blind estimates that approximately 0.03 % of newborn babies have a congenital cataract. In most cases there is no obvious cause, but there may be a family history of congenital cataract, or rarely the condition might relate to congenital rubella, toxoplasmosis or cytomegalovirus infections or a history of maternal drug therapy, particularly with steroids and thalidomide. Not all congenital cataracts require urgent surgery in newborns. The ophthalmologist will assess the size and density of the cataract, which may be tiny, and unilateral. If the baby has little sight, surgery may be carried out during the first month of life, so that the retina, optic nerves and brain are stimulated to develop the sense of vision, so that the child may develop as a sighted individual. Intraocular lenses may be implanted in babies, but lens calculations for children with a very small eye and aged less than 36 months have been found to result in large refractive errors (Tromans *et al.*, 2001). Spectacles or contact lenses may be used in the first instance.

Remember that a potential eye problem in a newborn is devastating news for the parents who will have been hoping for a 'perfect' baby. Often a thorough diagnosis of the problem cannot be made until the child has been examined under general anaesthesia, which is a risk-laden procedure for a newborn. The mother will still be recovering from the birth; her hormone levels are likely to be fluctuating and sleep may be lost due to night feeds. Both parents will need a lot of emotional and practical support from the staff.

Acquired cataracts

Symptoms

Symptoms of adult cataract include some of the following (remember that generally one eye is affected more than the other at first presentation):

- *Index myopia* as a result of the lens beginning to swell as the cataract develops. This causes improved near vision without spectacles ('second sight'). Increased visits to the optometrist may be necessary as visual acuity fluctuates. Eventually surgery becomes necessary.

- *Painless, blurred near and distant vision* due to decreased accommodation by the hardening lens.

- *Decreased colour appreciation* as the lens ages. It yellows and absorbs more short-wave light, so the patient tends to lose appreciation of blues and greens gradually, while becoming more aware of yellows and oranges.

Posterior subcapsular cataracts (in the cortex near the central posterior capsule) tend to cause visual symptoms earlier in their development due to involvement of the visual axis. Symptoms include *glare* and reduced vision under bright lighting conditions. For example, when driving at night the oncoming headlights of other cars can be particularly dazzling. For some working people who drive a lot, particularly in the dark (e.g. sales representatives) this can be extremely disabling.

The severity of sight impairment is assessed by use of a Snellen chart and by questioning the person about how their eyesight is affecting their daily activities. Surprisingly, some people who have fairly advanced cataracts on examination may have little difficulty in carrying out their normal activities. However, others may have surprising problems with only slight opacity of a lens. In many people, cataracts develop slowly over many years, and surgery may never be necessary.

To do ...

Find out more about visual function and coping. Why do some people have quite good visual acuity, but are still given cataract surgery?

Check the Eye Digest website for some of the answers.

You could also try to find out more about the VF-14. This is a visual function questionnaire that some eye units ask patients to complete prior to cataract consultation.

Predisposing factors in cataract development

These are:

- excessive exposure to ultraviolet light (e.g. from sunshine)
- a diet lacking in essential vitamins and minerals
- diabetes mellitus
- a strong family history of cataracts
- myopia
- recurrent attacks of uveitis
- conditions requiring the regular local or systemic use of steroids

- smoking (Raju *et al.*, 2006)
- ageing.

Ageing is the most significant factor leading to cataract formation.

Age-related cataracts

These are of three types.

Subcapsular cataracts

These may occur in the anterior or posterior sections of the lens. Typically, affected patients may be younger and particularly sensitive to headlights of oncoming cars and bright sunlight. These cataracts are generally central, and therefore can cause a dramatic reduction in vision as they develop.

Nuclear cataracts

Nuclear cataracts cause a general decrease in the transparency of the lens nucleus. They are associated with index myopia.

Cortical cataracts

These involve the lens cortex, which develops radial, wedge-shaped opacities. Sometimes they cause astigmatic type changes in the vision, and monocular diplopia.

Other types of acquired cataracts

Traumatic cataract

Traumatic cataract may be caused by:

- penetrating injury to the eye (e.g. industrial injury)
- blunt injury to the eye (e.g. boxing)
- electric shock and lightning (rare!)
- exposure to radiation (e.g. to treat tumours of the eye or face or total body irradiation for leukaemia).

You can read more about traumatic cataracts by checking Graham and Mulrooney (2009).

Metabolic cataract

An age-related cataract may develop earlier and progress more quickly in a person with type 1 or 2 diabetes. A diabetic cataract results from over-hydration of the lens, and appears as bilateral white 'snowflake-like' lens opacities. Sometimes an 'early' cataract is the first symptom of type 2 diabetes. Very rare metabolic disorders such as phenylketonuria or galactosaemia cause cataracts to develop in infants due to faulty body metabolism.

Drugs and cataract formation

Both systemic and topical steroids can cause cataracts. Children are more vulnerable than adults. A range of other drugs are implicated in cataract formation, but the benefits of receiving these treatments, as with steroids, generally far outweigh the risks.

Secondary complicated cataract

Secondary complicated cataract may develop as a result of some other optic disease. High myopia, retinitis pigmentosa, recurrent uveitis, chronic glaucoma, retinal and glaucoma surgery are all implicated in the formation of secondary cataract.

Epidemiology of cataracts

This area of study relates to the incidence, distribution, management and prevention of cataracts. Read the online article by Hammond (2000) on the epidemiology of cataracts.

To do ...

Start looking in the notes of younger patients, particularly at their medical histories, to see if there is any reason why they have developed an earlier cataract.

Make brief notes on an interesting cataract patient, maintaining confidentiality and focusing on their eye condition. Add them to your personal folder. Remember that the best learning occurs when you apply what you have learned in practice. Throughout your career you will build up a personal 'memory bank' of patients you have learned from.

Cataract maturity

Once the ophthalmologist has diagnosed the patient with a cataract, a note is made regarding its maturity and whether surgery may be carried out by a consultant, staff grade or specialist registrar. Consultants always aim to carry out the most complicated operations, which can make participating in their operating theatre lists particularly good learning experiences for all staff.

Immature cataract

Only part of the lens is opaque. Most cataract surgery is now undertaken at this stage.

Mature cataract

The whole lens is opaque and may be swollen (intumescent). If the lens takes up water it may cause a secondary glaucoma. A consultant would generally manage this case.

Hyper-mature cataract

The lens may become dehydrated due to escape of water from the lens, leaving an opaque lens and wrinkled capsule. Alternatively, the lens cortex may become soft and milky so that the nucleus sinks to the bottom of the capsule (a Morgagnian cataract). Lens matter may even leak out causing uveitis and secondary (phacolytic) glaucoma. This is a consultant case. Cataracts should normally be extracted before this situation arises. (Note that they are rare in UK society due to healthcare availability that is 'free' at the point of delivery.)

N.B. Traumatic cataract

Any break in the lens capsule following a traumatic injury is followed rapidly by cataract changes. As aqueous fluid seeps inside the lens capsule, a swollen (intumescent) lens develops. This may eventually result in an acute secondary glaucoma due to 'crowding' in the anterior chamber. This cataract will need to be removed promptly under consultant supervision. Ask the ophthalmologist if they wish to prescribe acetazolamide (Diamox™) prior to pupil dilatation. Do not dilate this patient too early prior to surgery because the intraocular pressure may rise quickly, causing acute preoperative complications.

One-stop cataract facility

An optician or GP may refer patients to the ophthalmic department. With a good referral letter, patients can be given a direct appointment to a one-stop cataract clinic. This arrangement has a number of advantages for the patient and the NHS as it helps to shorten waiting times, reduces the number of visits the patient has to make to the hospital, and facilitates improved patient assessment and preparation and speedier patient outcomes.

The patient visits for an ophthalmic assessment and sees the consultant to establish that cataract surgery is the right approach and whether any other eye problem is involved, such as advanced macular degeneration or a large retinal detachment. Once the consultant and patient have discussed the situation and potential visual outcome (particularly where a retinal anomaly is involved) and decided that cataract surgery is required, the pre-assessment nurse will obtain a mutually agreed date for the patient's surgery. All the eye measurements and preoperative assessments will be carried out and the patient returns home with a date for surgery, fully aware of what is going to happen to them and with all their immediate questions answered. A contact number should be provided for use if further questions or health changes occur or if the patient is unable to attend on the due date.

Preoperative preparation

To do ...

- Arrange to work with the pre-admission nurses.
- Ask patients about their cataract symptoms prior to surgery.
- Find out about the nurse's role in measuring for intraocular lenses.
- What steps are taken to ensure the measurements are accurate?
- What should the nurse do to prepare for the patient's admission when it is known that an unusual lens size will be required?
- Find out why some patients are unsuitable for local anaesthetic.

Then

- Ask if you can help in the ophthalmic day surgery ward for a morning so that you can learn about the immediate preoperative preparation for cataract surgery.

Preoperative assessment of the cataract patient

It is important to give a basic understanding of the cataract procedure and its possible complications and to talk about what to expect on the day of surgery. The nurse needs to be understanding and take into account the ability of the patient to instil eye-drops regularly postoperatively. Eye-drop instillation technique will be demonstrated, any difficulties will be discussed and use of appropriate eye-drop devices advised. If necessary, the patient may be given a bottle of artificial tears to take home to practise with. For patients who have difficulty manipulating eye-drop bottles, or who are unable to raise their arms sufficiently to instil drops, eye-drop administering devices are available.

Patients will also need to be told whether they may eat and drink prior to surgery. Those with diabetes mellitus will need an explanation as to how their diabetes will be managed under local or general anaesthetic. Patients on anticoagulants will need specific instructions regarding preoperative blood tests and whether or not to omit their medication. Clear verbal instructions should be given and any questions answered. All the information imparted should be accompanied by clear, accurate written information that the patient (and possibly their relatives or carers) can refer to later. A telephone contact number should be given, so that the patient can contact the clinic if they have further questions or their health status changes.

The preoperative assessment will also involve measurement of the patient's spectacle prescription using a focimeter and the measurement of both eyes using either the IOL Master™ or an A-scan machine.

Spectacle wear

It is important to record the prescription of distance, bifocal or varifocal spectacles by the patient and take an accurate history of when they first wore spectacles (Table 5.1). You will need this information to determine the accuracy of your intraocular lens measurements.

Table 5.1 *Age at first spectacles*

Hypermetropia	Lifelong/spherical lens (+) Early reading glasses needed
Myopia	Lifelong/spherical lens (–) Later life only (probably index myopia)
Presbyopia	Spherical lens (+)

Blurred near vision is commonly evident after the age of 40. This is due to the reduction in the power of accommodation.

Electronic focimeter/lens analyser

This machine is designed to measure all types of spectacle lenses. The basic operation is menu-driven by icons marked on the screen. By touching the button of the appropriate icon, the screen will take you to the menu selection or execute a command. The machine will automatically read the lens, and the data can then be stored in the memory. There are two programmes for measuring spectacle lenses – one for single vision lenses and one for bifocal or varifocal lenses.

Positioning the spectacles

It is important that the spectacles are placed correctly on the machine. They must be positioned with the arms down, with the lens to be measured lying over the analysing lens head. The bridge of the spectacles should be against the nose slider, which acts as an artificial nose to ensure the spectacles are positioned correctly; it also tells the analyser which side of the spectacles is being measured.

The lower edges of the spectacle frames should be touching the lens table. The lens table moves to accommodate spectacles of varying size. To move the lens table, either use the adjustment handle, or push or pull it into position. It is important that this is done to ensure that the spectacles are straight when measured. If they are not, the lens axis measured on the spectacles will be altered. An accurate focimetry reading recorded by a nurse or technician is essential – there is some potential for the patient's postoperative astigmatism to be reduced because the surgeon may rely on the axis of the patient's preoperative prescription to decide where to make his or her incision into the eye.

Once the spectacles are in the correct position on the focimeter (Fig. 5.1), the lens clamp can be used to stabilise the lenses during measurement. When the focimeter detects a lens, it will show a cursor that you can use to centre the lens to produce an accurate reading. Most modern machines also print out the reading for you. The patient's name should be written on it immediately, and it should be stapled to their notes securely.

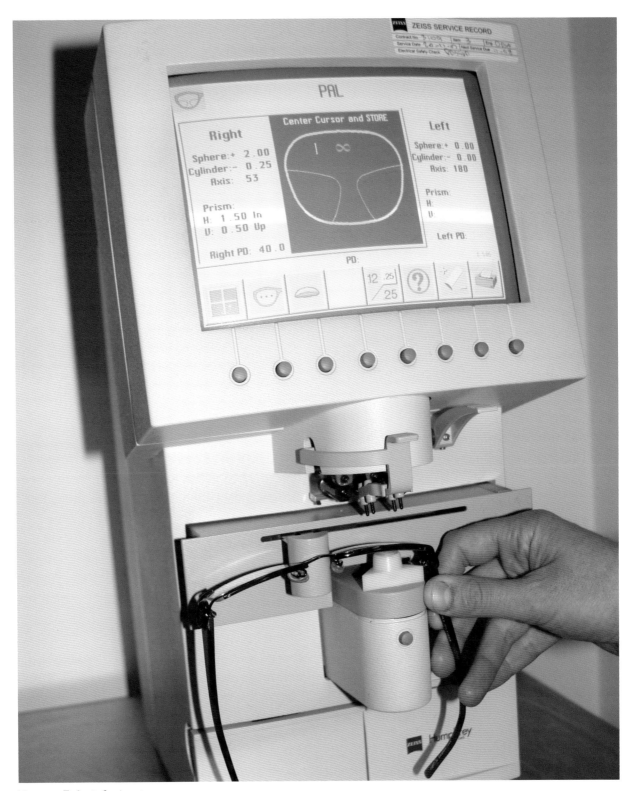

Figure 5.1 *A focimeter*
© Samantha Hartley, Ophthalmic Photographer, Royal Bournemouth Hospital, UK.

To do ...

Make sure you have read Chapter 3 carefully and completed the activities associated with it. You may need to re-visit it in order to understand some of the information below.

Biometry

Biometry is a very wide term that relates to the application of statistical mathematical data to biological data to produce measurements. It can therefore be applied to any part of the body, but in ophthalmology it refers to eye measurements. The measurements that particularly concern us are discussed below. They refer to obtaining data that will enable the fitting of a prescription intraocular lens to enable clear vision for a patient following cataract surgery.

Axial length of the eye – understanding its significance

The refractive power of the eye is a combination of the corneal power (keratometry), the lens power, and the axial length of the eye. If these are in balance, no spectacle lenses are necessary for distance vision because light can be focused on the retina. In most people, the average axial length of the eye measured from the posterior corneal surface to the vitreoretinal interface is about 23 mm.

If light comes to a focus at a point *behind* the retina, the eye is hypermetropic (long-sighted, requiring + lenses). This is usually due to a short axial length. In this instance, axial length is around 21 mm or below.

If however, the light comes to a focus *in front of* the retina, the eye is myopic (short-sighted, requiring – lenses). This is usually due to a long axial length if spectacles have been worn from a young age. This person's axial length is usually about 26 mm.

Many eyes become increasingly myopic as a result of a nuclear cataract that increases the curvature of the natural lens. Reading spectacles will only have become necessary in the patient's middle years, and these eyes have a normal axial length.

The IOL Master™

This machine is used to record measurements from a patient's eyes using a laser light. It measures the curvatures of the cornea in two meridians (written as K1 and K2) and the length of the eye (axial length). These two readings are used by the IOL Master™ (Fig. 5.2) to calculate the dioptric power of the lens implant required taking into account the A constant of the proposed implant. The A constant may be defined as a numerical calculation based on the optical design and material of the implant and the position in which it is to be placed within the eye. All lens styles and makes will have slightly different A constants, and the biometry reading from the IOL Master™ will normally be calculated on the A constant of the lenses purchased by the department, which has been recorded within the IOL Master™. If a different lens is to be used, the lens power will need to be re-calculated by altering the settings of the IOL Master™.

It is important to explain the biometry procedure to the patient, as the machine requires both cooperation and reasonable concentration. The nurse must first ensure that the patient is in a comfortable position in their chair, with their head in the frame of the machine throughout the procedure. The height adjuster within the head frame must be used to ensure that the patient's eyes are aligned with the markers at either side of the frame. The patient must concentrate on looking at the bright light in the machine. They can blink, but they must keep their eyes as still as possible.

The advantage of the IOL Master™ is that no part of the apparatus touches the eye, and so (provided the machine is cleaned between patients) there is little possibility of transmitting an infection. Because the machine uses laser interferometry, its readings have potentially greater precision than with ultrasound (an A-scan), and it can measure the corneal vertex through to the retinal pigment epithelium to +/– 0.02 mm. Look at the axial length (AL) display for a high SNR (signal to noise ratio) whereby an SNR of more than 2 is a good reading. A low SNR is likely to indicate poor alignment of the machine to the patient's eye, a dense cataract, poor fixation by the patient or a refractive error possibly in excess of 6 dioptres, or even, very rarely, retinal pathology.

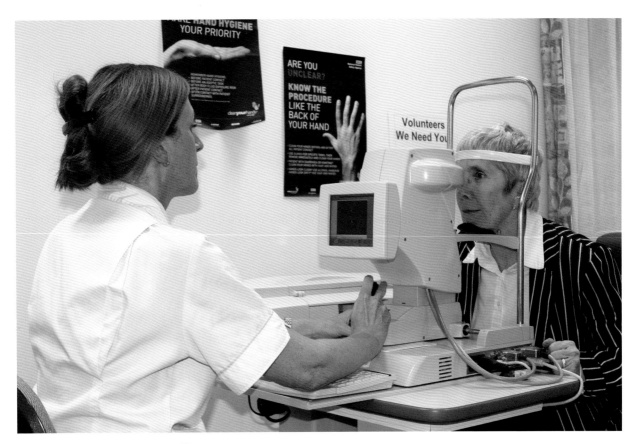

Figure 5.2 *The IOL Master*™ © Samantha Hartley, Ophthalmic Photographer, Royal Bournemouth Hospital, UK.

Asbury and Ramamurthy (2006) found that the outcome of cataract surgery will result in at least 80% of eyes being within 1 dioptre of the desired focus following surgery. Most UK ophthalmic units audit their surgical outcomes.

Even though most readings are obtained from the automated IOL Master™, it is of critical importance that a skilled biometrist – a nurse or PAM (profession allied to medicine) – should always be available to check any inconsistent scans, re-scan the patient or to double check with the A-scan machine.

There are a number of possible problems with the IOL Master™; sometimes it is not possible to obtain readings due to:

- Dense cataract: The light beam in the machine cannot penetrate through the cataract to obtain a reading.
- Poor keratometry readings: These may be due to dry eye (in the first instance ask the patient to blink a few times or even lubricate the eye using hydroxyethyl cellulose (hypromellose drops), or corneal scarring.
- Variable axial length reading: This may be due to previous retinal surgery (scleral band or vitrectomy) or an amblyopic eye.

 You can read more about the IOL Master™ and download an IOL Master™ manual at the Doctor Hill website.

Check to see if your eye department has written a biometry protocol. If not, check whether one is available on the internet – and read it. It could help you with your learning in practice.

To do ...

Find out how important the signal to noise ratio (SNR) is in obtaining an accurate reading.

Find some of the names of other calculation formulas that can be used in the IOL Master™.

Who is responsible for any changes in the settings of this machine?

How might the accuracy of measurements be audited?

The A-scan machine

This machine measures the axial length of the eye using an ultrasound method. It is usually resorted to when a patient has a cataract that is too dense to permit measurement by the IOL Master™. Using the A-scan, the eye will be touched by the operator with a blunt pencil-like probe. Explanation of the technique is essential because complete patient cooperation is needed.

Local anaesthetic eye-drops must be instilled to numb the cornea. The patient must focus their eyes straight ahead, then the probe is placed very gently on the centre of the cornea. The probe must break the tear film of the eye, but not bend the cornea, as this would shorten the axial length of the eye. An ultrasound signal passes into the eye and bounces back, so recording the axial length of the eye.

This can be a less accurate way of measuring the eye because:

- the machine makes assumptions about the density of the cataract, which varies from patient to patient
- the probe can be pressed too heavily on the cornea, bending the cornea and shortening the readings
- the probe may be poorly positioned
- the patient may not cooperate.

Once the measurements have been satisfactorily obtained from the A-scan, they can be entered into the IOL Master™. Together with the K1 and K2 readings, the machine will process the information and calculate the implant size required for the patient.

An excellent article about the use of the A-scan has been published by Asbury and Ramamurthy (2006) and is available at via the National Library for Health.

Table 5.2 relates to spectacle wear throughout adult life. High index myopia may account for discrepancies, which is why it is important to know:

- Whether spectacles have been worn for most of the person's life.
- Whether the optometrist's referral letter mentions any difficulty in keeping up with the patient's increasing refractive changes.
- Whether spectacles were prescribed relatively recently for index myopia.

Table 5.2 *Checking your readings by comparing biometry readings with spectacle prescriptions*

Distance glasses	Expected intraocular lens power
+ 3.00 Dioptre	+ 25–26 Dioptre
No spectacles	+ 21–22
−1.5	+ 19–20
−3	+ 18
−6	+ 15–18
−10	+ 10–14
−20	No IOL

Competence in practice

Gaining a satisfactory amount of knowledge to work unsupervised in the preoperative preparation of cataract patients (a highly significant role within ophthalmology) can take a nurse quite a long time, even if he or she has a recognised ophthalmic qualification. The value of attending biometry study days and repeated practice in terms of developing accuracy in biometry measurements has been recognised by two national biometry audits by Gale *et al.* (2004; 2006). These two studies also point out that nurses are now responsible for 67% of all biometry measurements in the UK.

Intraoperative care

Intraoperative care is studied in Chapter 6. To make sure that good relationships are maintained between the cataract/day surgery department and the ophthalmic theatre, relevant information must be exchanged promptly about patient concerns and comfort needs. For example, an elderly woman with severe kyphosis will need expert help from theatre staff and take extra time to position adequately for surgery. A patient with claustrophobia may be reassured by 'practicing' with the theatre drapes or require a different style of draping. Preoperative staff must be aware of unusual lens measurements or styles that may be required for a patient. When an unusual lens strength or style is required for a specific patient, ensure that the ophthalmic theatre staff are given the opportunity to check their stock prior to the patient's admission, as it may be necessary to order a lens for such a patient. This will maintain an efficient service, avoid unnecessary patient cancellations and maintain good interdepartmental relationships.

References and further reading

Asbury, N. and Ramamurthy, B. (2006). How to avoid mistakes in biometry. *Community Eye Health Journal* 19(60), 70–71.

Gale, R., Saha, N. and Johnston, R. (2004). National Biometry Audit. *Eye*, 18, 63–66.

Gale, R., Saha, N. and Johnston, R. (2006). National Biometry Audit 2. *Eye*, 20, 25–27.

Graham, R. and Mulrooney, B. (2009). Cataract, traumatic. Available at: http://emedicine.medscape.com/article/1211083-overview (last accessed August 2009).

Hammond, C. (2000). The epidemiology of cataracts. *Optometry Today*, February 9, 24–28. Available at: http://www.otmagazine.co.uk/articles.php?year=2001.

Raju, P., George, R., Ramesh, S., Arvind, H., Baskaran, M. and Vijaya, L. (2006). The influence of tobacco use on cataract development. *British Journal of Ophthalmology*, 90, 1374–77.

Tromans, C., Haig, P., Biswas, S. and Lloyd, R. (2001). Accuracy of intraocular lens power calculation in paediatric cataract surgery. *British Journal of Ophthalmology*, 85(8), 939–41.

Useful web resources

Doctor Hill
www.doctor-hill.com/IOL Master_main.htm
Information about optical biometry.

National Library for Health
www.library.nhs.uk/

Optometry Today
http://www.optometry.co.uk/

Optician Online
http://www.opticianonline.net/Home/Default.aspx
Look for Malhotra's article on the ageing lens and classification of cataracts.

Royal National Institute for the Blind
http://www.rnib.org.uk/xpedio/groups/public/documents/PublicWebsite/public_rnib003644.hcsp

The Eye Digest
http://www.ageingeye.net/.
More on the symptoms of cataract.

SELF TEST answers on page 204

1. What is index myopia caused by?

2. Why do posterior subcapsular cataracts tend to cause earlier visual symptoms?

3. A person with diabetes might develop what kind of cataract beginning with the letter 'm'?

4. Which group of drugs is particularly associated with cataract development?

5. What word beginning with 'i' describes a traumatic cataract with a swollen lens?

6. Name the machine used to measure spectacle lenses in clinic.

7. The refractive power of the eye is measured on the IOL Master™ in the cataract clinic using three elements. What are these?

8. What is the axial length of most eyes?

9. Would a person with an axial length of 21 mm or below be myopic or hypermetropic?

Chapter 6

Intraoperative management of cataract patients

Dorothy Field

For people who work in ophthalmic theatres, cataract surgery continues to be a fascination in terms of the variety of patients undergoing the procedure, the types of cataracts encountered, and the continued streamlining of ophthalmic technique and instrumentation. The quality of the staff supporting the patients and surgeons makes a great contribution to the patient's eventual visual outcome. This chapter has been designed to help new theatre staff to understand a little more about what happens and why it happens, and to learn some of the associated vocabulary. Similarly, it is hoped that those with responsibilities lying outside the theatre will understand why cataract surgery is sometimes complex and more time consuming for their patients. Staff employed in preoperative and postoperative cataract clinics should be given a reasonable amount of time to observe ophthalmic surgery in order to provide excellent preoperative patient preparation and to understand some of the potential complexities of this highly skilled form of surgery.

To do ...

Arrange to spend time in the eye theatre to observe some of the practices and procedures below.

Patient position

Given that most cataract surgery is carried out under local anaesthetic, much consideration should be given to the patient's warmth and comfort during the procedure. Table padding may be necessary for people with joint and spinal problems. Many eye units place a pillow under the patient's knees to relieve stress on the spine and pressure on the heels for the short duration of the surgery. Nervous patients may appreciate having their hand held (Chang, 2001) but do ask the

63

patient first! People with advanced psychoprophylactic coping strategies may find that this destroys the coping mechanisms that they have developed.

Local anaesthesia

Ideal conditions for a surgeon undertaking cataract surgery include the absence of painful sensations for the patient, the inability of the patient to move the eye (akinesia) and the inability to squeeze the eyelids shut. The lowest possible risk of complications and postoperative pain are significant considerations, as are ease of use and speed of administration for the maintenance of an efficient patient-focused service.

Monitoring during local anaesthesia

The Royal College of Ophthalmologists Cataract Surgery Guidelines state in section 6.5.2 that systemic adverse events have been reported in all forms of anaesthesia during cataract surgery, including topical.

Section 6.7.1 of the guidelines recommends starting patient monitoring before administration of the local anaesthetic, and throughout the procedure.

Oculocardiac reflex (the Aschner phenomenon)

Tension on the extraocular muscles or pressure on the eyeball can cause bradycardia, junctional rhythm, or even asystole (oculocardiac reflex). This is why monitoring of all ophthalmic patients during procedures is recommended and it is one of the main reasons for the Royal College of Ophthalmologists' recommendation that an anaesthetist should attend ophthalmic operating lists. Babies and young children are particularly at risk from this problem during squint surgery. If there is a change in the pulse rate or ECG, the anaesthetist will ask the ophthalmologist to release tension on the muscle or pressure on the eye immediately. Atropine may be used to prevent or treat the problem.

The afferent pathway of this stimulus is via the ciliary ganglion to the ophthalmic division of the trigeminal nerve to the Gasserian ganglion. These afferent pathways synapse with the visceral motor nucleus of the vagus nerve in the brainstem. The efferent message is carried back via the vagus nerve to the medulla of the heart, leading to decreased output from the sinoatrial node, causing bradycardia. There is a small possibility that the administration of a local anaesthetic around the eye could trigger this phenomenon.

Local anaesthetic injections

Sub-Tenon's injection. This is carried out after topical anaesthetic drops have been instilled. A small opening is made into the conjunctiva that lies over the medial and inferior rectus, using dissecting scissors. A blunt cannula is carefully introduced into this space, and local anaesthetic solution injected. Of all the injection methods for producing local anaesthesia, this is currently the most popular, carrying fewer of the risks associated with retrobulbar or peribulbar injections. Administration of the injection following the eye-drops is pain free. The amount of akinesia produced is variable.

Retrobulbar injection. This carries a number of rare, but serious, risks and is now rarely used for cataract surgery. Occasionally it is used prior to laser photocoagulation. It involves passing a needle along the floor of the orbit to deposit local anaesthetic around the ciliary ganglion. When accurately placed, this technique provides excellent local anaesthesia and renders the patient incapable of moving the eye or squeezing the eyelids together during surgery.

Peribulbar injection/s. Administered on the temporal side of the orbit, into the extraconal space, the needle is not inserted as deeply as for the retrobulbar injection. This is considered to carry fewer risks of complication. Expert administration produces good akinesia.

Topical anaesthesia

This popular method of anaesthesia has been termed the 'vocal local' because of the high level of patient preparation required before surgery, and because it is essential that the patient complies with the surgeon's instructions to keep looking at the microscope light throughout the procedure and avoid squeezing the muscles around the eye as the local anaesthetic drops will produce no akinesia.

Drops of tetracaine 1% (amethocaine) or some other local anaesthetic instilled into the upper and lower fornices of the eye are now frequently used for uncomplicated cataract extractions in compliant patients. The method produces a good level of analgesia, but any manipulation of the iris, anterior chamber distension and intraocular lens insertion can be uncomfortable. It is for this reason occasionally that intracameral analgesia is necessary during surgery, whereby local anaesthetic is introduced directly into the eye.

The topical method of producing local anaesthesia by instilling eye-drops is popular with patients who are (understandably) nervous of injections in the vicinity of the eye. It is also reasonably risk-free, quick and cheap. Obviously if surgery is likely to be lengthy or complicated, or if the patient is very nervous, then local anaesthetic injection with sedation or general anaesthesia would be considered.

Preparing for surgery

A small pupil can make surgery very difficult, so it is important that the staff preparing the patient administer and monitor the effects of the prescribed dilating drops. If the pupil is not dilating well, a message should be sent to the surgeon prior to the commencement of surgery. There are a variety of devices such as hooks and rings that the surgeon may require to stretch the pupil open. Make sure that you investigate the types your theatre stocks, and observe them in use at the first available opportunity. Use of an iris ring or hooks will leave the pupil unreactive following surgery.

Scrub and circulating staff should be aware of the surgeon's preferences for such supplementary equipment during complicated surgery and either anticipate their need or be able to produce what is required quickly and quietly.

Some eye units also use preoperative diclofenac drops to counteract surgically induced miosis. The phaco-irrigation bag may contain epinephrine 1:1,000,000 for the same reason (Liou and Yang, 1998).

Draping the patient

The patient's face and the upper part of his or her body will be well covered to reduce the risk of intraocular infection. Reassurance is essential as pulse and respiration often increase at this time. Normally the surgical drape is arranged over an anaesthetic screen so that it is not resting directly on the patient's face. Staff must ensure that the patient has an adequate oxygen supply because the draping towels are relatively impervious, and there is a danger of a carbon dioxide build-up beneath them (Risdale and Geraghty, 1999). This is one of the reasons for using a pulse oximeter during surgery.

Ophthalmic theatre staff behaviour

All staff within the eye theatre should remember that the patient, particularly when surgery is carried out under topical anaesthesia, has to concentrate on staying still, and keeping his or her eye still. Sudden noises and raised voices should be avoided at all times, particularly when complications are encountered.

Only the surgeon should speak directly to the patient while surgery is in progress. If you are hand-holding for a patient who is communicating signs of distress, speak to the scrub person who will communicate with the surgeon at an appropriate moment. Do not speak to the patient yourself because this may cause them to move their head – the scrub person should know if the surgeon (who probably has a surgical instrument in the patient's eye) is carrying out a particularly delicate process and will choose the first suitable opportunity to pass the message on. The surgeon will then speak to the patient directly when there is no instrument in the eye. Similarly, if you are 'circulating' in theatre, it is important to pass any messages for the surgeon to the scrub person, who will pass your message to the surgeon at a suitable moment.

Are patients able to see what is happening during cataract surgery?

The move towards topical anaesthesia, which does not affect optic nerve function, has brought increasing concerns about patients' visual awareness. Reassuringly, the patient information leaflet *Understanding Cataracts* produced by the Royal College of Ophthalmologists (2001) states 'you may vaguely see some signs of movement, but no details of the operation.' A study set up by Chung *et al.* (2004) compared patients' experiences under retrobulbar anaesthesia and topical anaesthesia. A group of 76 patients were studied, of whom 41 were in the retrobulbar group and 35 in the topical group. Two patients in the retrobulbar group had no light perception throughout surgery. No patient in the topical group experienced loss of light perception. During surgery, 73% of all patients perceived colour changes. Patients in both groups saw waves, and some of the topical group saw a rectangular moving object at some stages in the surgery.

The instruments

Wadood and Dhillon (2002) make a number of recommendations regarding management of the surgical trolley and the passing of ophthalmic instruments. Their article is recommended reading. Key standards for the scrub person include only touching the handles of instruments that are going to be used inside the eye, and being extremely careful to correctly secure cannulae to syringes and phaco-emulsification hand-pieces. Despite warnings within the published literature (e.g. Wiggins and Uwaydat, 2008), cannulae continue to detach from syringes during ocular surgery, sometimes causing quite severe injuries to patients' eyes.

The scrub person's ophthalmic responsibilities

- Check the correct eye with a valid consent form.
- Check the lens size, make and expiry date.
- Ensure all staff are aware of any relevant patient allergies, including to eye-drops.
- Be responsible for checking all fluids entering the eye during surgery.
- Ensure that the phaco machine is set to the surgeon's requirements throughout surgery.

Scrub practitioners need to know how the lens-delivery systems (introducers) used in their theatre suite for folding lenses work, and which lens they are used for. They should have practised folding lenses and have been assessed as competent.

Inexperienced scrub practitioners must be well supported until they are capable of managing the wide range of challenges that occur during ophthalmic surgery.

Phaco-emulsification of cataract

Phaco-emulsification (also known simply as 'phaco') is a means of liquefying solid matter using high-frequency sound waves. Within ophthalmology, a 'phaco machine' is used to deliver sound waves at the correct frequency to liquefy lens material and provide a stream of a balanced salt solution to cool the operating end of the hand-piece, to wash and suck out cellular debris from the lens capsule and to maintain a constant pressure within the eye. The machine is set up to the ophthalmologist's requirements by the theatre team, and is operated by the surgeon using foot controls (the 'phaco pedal'). It has become the most common approach to cataract surgery in the UK.

Phaco cataract surgery

Phaco cataract surgery is approached as follows. A small (side port) incision is made in the cornea. The surgeon can therefore use a second instrument for manipulation purposes during the surgery. Viscoelastic gel is injected into the eye to maintain the shape of the anterior chamber, to provide a 'space' for the surgeon to operate in and protect the delicate endothelial cells on the under surface of the cornea.

Then a second, larger corneal incision is made into the anterior chamber of the eye (a scleral 'tunnel' approach is sometimes used instead). The surgeon uses a sharp instrument to begin to tear a tiny flap in the anterior capsular membrane, which covers the anterior surface of the lens. With the utmost care, capsulorhexis forceps are used to tear this flap carefully into a complete circle. This tear is called the capsulorhexis.

The lens nucleus within the soft lens matter is mobilised by hydrodissection. It is achieved by injecting a small quantity of balanced salt solution into the capsular bag. The surgeon checks that the nucleus will rotate within the capsular bag.

Phaco-emulsification uses high-frequency sound waves to break up the hard nucleus of the lens. Some surgeons use a chopping technique, and others make deep grooves to divide the lens into quarters before finally carving up and aspirating the pieces. The remnants of the lens cortex are aspirated from the lens 'bag' using the irrigating and aspiration (I/A) handpiece.

Viscoelastic is injected into the capsular bag to expand it and facilitate the implantation of the intraocular lens. After double-checking the prescription with the surgeon, the lens is implanted into the eye and rotated into the correct position within the capsular bag. The viscoelastic is removed using the I/A and the anterior chamber is re-formed using balanced salt solution. Finally, the surgeon checks for any wound leaks, and that the intraocular pressure is around normal, by applying gentle pressure to the cornea.

Possible intraoperative problems

Expulsive haemorrhage

This rare complication can occur during any type of intraocular surgery. As the incision is made into the eye, the sudden reduction in eye pressure may lead to a spontaneous tear and haemorrhage from a ciliary artery. Hypertension, a myopic eye (increased axial length – sometimes referred to as a bulgy eye) and raised intraocular pressure are among many possible causes of this phenomenon.

Expulsive haemorrhage

Expulsive haemorrhage is an emergency. The surgeon must discontinue surgery immediately and close the wound to prevent the eye contents being prolapsed through the incision.

Phaco self-sealing wounds are considered safer than the previous methods of cataract surgery because the surgeon can immediately terminate the procedure in the event of an expulsive haemorrhage.

Corneal decompensation

In eyes with Fuchs' dystrophy, for example, corneal decompensation may occur in the postoperative period due to the trauma of cataract surgery. Viscoelastic solution will help to protect the cells of the corneal endothelium during surgery.

Floppy iris syndrome

This tends to be a problem in patients receiving tamsulosin (Flomax™) although it does not affect all these patients. Chadha *et al.* (2006) found that 57% of patients were affected in their study. Friedman (2007) describes how this condition can lead to poor preoperative pupil dilatation, and an iris that 'billows' and prolapses readily during surgery. He notes that this increases the possibility of trauma to the iris, posterior capsule rupture and vitreous loss. Most ophthalmologists have worked out their personal strategies for dealing with this problem, but Friedman (2007) gives an overview of the different devices that can be used to manage it.

Weakness of the lens zonules

This may be a problem particularly as a result of a pre-existing condition such as pseudexfoliation or Marfan syndrome. Occasionally a few zonules are broken before surgery commences. The pressure exerted on the capsule during the phaco-emulsification procedure may cause the lens to become unstable. (This is a consultant case!) At worst, the complete lens may fall back into the vitreous. It is then a vitreoretinal surgeon's job to remove it.

White cataract

A 'white' cataract is sometimes referred to by ophthalmologists. It is a hyper-mature cataract, which makes it very difficult to see and control the capsulorhexis tear.

 See Cataract and Refractive Surgery Today for a review of this condition.

The scrub person will on request prepare either trypan blue (Vision Blue) or indocyanine green dye. The scrub person may also require two or three extra 2 mL syringes. The surgeon will probably ask for the theatre lights to be dimmed to help visualise the structures.

Brown cataract

A 'brown' cataract is a very advanced cataract with a very hard brown nucleus. It takes a long time to break up with the phaco apparatus.

Problems with the capsulorhexis

These are a major complication. If the tear gets out of control it may extend into the posterior capsule. If the tear in the posterior capsule is extensive, there is a danger of the lens nucleus falling back into the vitreous ('dropped nucleus'). In order to avoid this complication and to try to control a wayward tear, the surgeon may ask for Ong scissors.

A hole in the posterior capsule can occur at most stages of cataract surgery. The infusion bag on the phaco machine will be lowered in order to reduce the pressure of fluid going into the eye in an attempt to prevent the tear increasing. There is a danger of losing the lens nucleus into the vitreous, and a 21 G needle (long orange) may be called for immediately to 'spear' the nucleus. If the surgeon is unable to prevent this happening, the cataract surgery will be completed with possibly no lens implant or an anterior chamber implant, or abandoned. The patient will be referred to a vitreoretinal surgeon so that any fragments of lens nucleus in the vitreous must be removed, as untreated they will cause posterior uveitis. You can read more about this from the surgeon's point of view in Chang (2001).

Vitreous prolapse into the anterior chamber may result from a tear in the posterior capsule. In order to avoid the danger of vitreous strands being caught up in the phaco wound and causing a retinal detachment later (see Chapter 11), an anterior vitrectomy will be required to remove and chop away any vitreous strands from the anterior chamber.

Patients and staff do not always understand that during cataract surgery unforeseen difficulties may occur for the most experienced surgeon during what at first sight appears to be straightforward surgery. It is a testament to the surgeons' skill and alertness and quick-thinking professional theatre staff that the vast majority of patients enjoy a satisfactory outcome.

The dependence of consultant ophthalmologists on experienced ophthalmic scrub staff during complicated surgery is emphasised by Baylis *et al.* (2006). Wadood and Dhillon (2002) who are both ophthalmologists also acknowledge 'the heavy dependence of the surgeon on a close, almost telepathic understanding between scrub person and surgeon, whose dual focus should be on the patient's well-being in general, and the intraocular procedure in particular'. The theatre suite they work in has drafted a local policy on the role of the scrub person acting as first assistant to the surgeon in phaco-emulsification surgery. This includes education and instruction by medical and nursing staff and guidelines for good practice. Before a registered practitioner takes up the dual role of scrub person and first assistant in their department, they have to demonstrate clinical competence and practical proficiency in six cases, working with senior surgeons. Wadood and Dhillon (2002) also recommend that practitioners should attend the phaco-emulsification courses run for them by ophthalmic supply companies.

Whether you work in the operating theatre or not, you are recommended to follow up the information in this chapter, and to strive for a better understanding of what can happen during both routine and complex surgery, as this can affect the patient's visual prognosis and the length and type of follow-up required. This will be discussed at length in the following chapter.

References and further reading

Baylis, O., Adams, W., Allen, D. and Fraser, S. (2006). Do variations in the theatre team have an impact on the incidence of complications? *BMC Ophthalmology*, 6, 13.

Chadha, V., Borooah, S., Tey, A., Styles, C. and Singh, J. (2006). Floppy iris behaviour during cataract surgery. *British Journal of Ophthalmology*, 91, 40–42.

Chang, D.F. (2001). How to avoid a dropped nucleus. *Cataract and Refractive Surgery Today*. Available at: http://www.crstodayarchive.com/03_archive/1101/archive_1_1101_11.html (last accessed June 2009).

Chang, S. (2001). The conceptual structure of physical touch in caring. *Journal of Advanced Nursing*, 33(6) 820–27.

Chung, F., Lai, J. and Lam, D. (2004). Visual sensation during phaco-emulsification using topical and regional anaesthesia. *Journal of Cataract and Refractive Surgery*, February, 31(10)444–48.

Department of Health (1999). *Focus on Cataract*. Available at: http://www.institute.nhs.uk/option,com_joomcart/Itemid,26/main_page,document_product_info/products_id,388.html (last accessed August 2009).

Friedman, N. (2007). Management of IFIS (intraoperative floppy iris syndrome). Available at: http://www.ophthalmologyweb.com/Spotlight.aspx?spid=23&aid=291 (last accessed August 2009).

Liou, S. and Yang, C. (1998). The effect of intracameral adrenaline infusion on pupil size during phaco-emulsification. *Journal of Ocular Pharmacology and Therapeutics* 14(4), 357–61.

Newman, D. (2000). Visual experience during phaco-emulsification cataract surgery with topical anaesthesia. *British Journal of Ophthalmology*, 84, 13–15.

Noble, B. and Simmons, I. (2001). *Complications of Cataract Surgery*. Oxford: Butterworth Heinemann.

Oscher, R. and Oscher, J. (2009). Confronting the white cataract. Available at: http://crstodayarchive.com/03_archive/1103/13.html (last accessed August 2009).

Risdale, J. and Geraghty, I. (1999). Oxygenation of patients undergoing ophthalmic surgery under local anaesthesia. *Anaesthesia*, 52(5), 492.

Royal College of Ophthalmologists (2001). *Understanding cataracts*. Available at: http://www.rcophth.ac.uk/docs/college/patientinfo/UnderstandingCataracts.pdf (last accessed August 2009).

Royal College of Ophthalmologists (2007). *Cataract Surgery Guidelines*. Available at: http://www.rcophth.ac.uk/docs/publications/published-guidelines/FinalVersionGuidelinesApril2007Updated.pdf (last accessed August 2009).

Tromans, C., Haig, P., Biswas, S. and Lloyd, R. (2001). Accuracy of intraocular lens power calculation in paediatric cataract surgery. *British Journal of Ophthalmology*, 85(8), 939–41.

Wadood, A. and Dhillon B. (2002). The role of the ophthalmic theatre nurse in phaco-emulsification surgery. *Ophthalmic Nursing* 6(3), 25–27.

Wiggins, M. and Uwaydat, S. (2008). Cannula ejection into the cornea during wound hydration. *British Journal of Ophthalmology*, 92, 181.

Useful web resources

AOL Video
http://video.aol.com/video-search/tag/pods
A huge range of video clips available. Type in exactly which aspect of surgery you wish to see, e.g. 'pupil expansion ring' and make your choice.

British Journal of Ophthalmology (BJO)
http://bjo.bmj.com/

Free Educational Publications International
www.eyepodvideo.org
About 30 ophthalmic surgical videos for viewing.

Good Hope Hospital Eye Department
http://www.goodhope.org.uk/departments/eyedept/

MedRounds
http://www.medrounds.org/
Lots of useful resources including 'video pods' which explore various aspects of surgery.

SELF TEST Answers on page 204

1. Tension on the extraocular muscles can cause bradycardia or even asystole. What is this called?

2. Which drug may be required in the treatment of the above syndrome?

3. Name two injection anaesthetic approaches that might be used for intraocular surgery.

4. The 'vocal local' is a description occasionally used for what approach to cataract surgery? Why is this so?

5. What are diclofenac eye-drops sometimes used preoperatively to counteract?

6. The phaco irrigation bag may contain epinephrine 1:1,000,000. Why?

7. Why must the theatre staff ensure that the patient's oxygen levels are monitored?

8. Who is the only person who may speak to the patient while surgery is in progress?

9. What is a capsulorhexis?

10. What is hydrodissection used for?

11. What two things might a hole in the capsular bag lead to?

Chapter 7

Postoperative cataract care

Claire Adams, Pauline Haley and Dorothy Field

This chapter covers examination of eyes soon after surgery, at follow-up and discharge as well as the value and limitations of giving advice over the telephone.

Same-day complications of cataract

A patient may get distressed if his or her eye is watering after surgery, and when they dry their face with a tissue there is a faint tinge of blood in the tears. This is generally because there is a tiny bleed from a conjunctival vessel. It is nothing to worry about so just reassure the patient.

If the patient has had regional anaesthesia with a retrobulbar or peribulbar injection, they may complain of double vision. This is because the patient still has akinesia; the external ocular muscles are paralysed and the eyes are not working together. A related temporary loss of the ability to blink may lead to corneal exposure with resulting pain as the sensation returns. The surgical team may pad the eye in theatre if these two symptoms are likely to occur.

A corneal abrasion may result from the patient opening the operated eye under an inadequately applied eye pad. Sometimes chloramphenicol eye ointment is used instead of a pad to coat the eye until the patient is able to blink again. Reassure the patient that while uncomfortable, the problem is not serious.

If the viscoelastic used during surgery is not sufficiently well removed or there is other debris within the anterior chamber, the intraocular pressure may rise causing acute eye pain. Patients often complain of a little pain after surgery. This is normal, and you should expect that it would be relieved with paracetamol 1g. If the pain becomes worse rather than better, an experienced nurse should (having cleansed their hands) remove the eye shield and check the patient's cornea with a torch or inspect the eye using a slit lamp. If the cornea is hazy, then it is likely that the pressure is raised, and the ophthalmologist needs to be informed urgently.

Postoperative reviews

These days it is not generally considered necessary to review the patient's eye routinely on the first postoperative day (Dinkaran et al., 2000; Tinley et al., 2003). Patients are generally given one outpatient appointment at 2 or 4 weeks post surgery. It is normal for patients and relatives to be counselled at their pre-admission visit and on discharge from the day-care unit regarding care of the eye on discharge. All verbal information should be reinforced with brief written advice.

General advice should include:

- simple analgesia
- hair washing
- gradual return to normal activities
- spectacle wearing.

Specific advice should include:

- removal of cartella shield and gentle eye bathing on first postoperative morning
- storage and instillation of eye-drops.

Also give advice on who to contact should any of the following flagged symptoms occur.

 Severe pain in the eye and brow area that is not alleviated by paracetamol 1g, particularly if accompanied by nausea and vomiting (which could indicate a rise in intraocular pressure).

 Vision from the operated eye on the first postoperative day is non-existent or is worse than it was preoperatively.

 Vision, which was initially satisfactory, begins to deteriorate slightly.

 There is a sticky discharge.

 The eye is stinging and watering.

 Double vision persists by the second day.

The Department of Health identified the following as the main complications of phaco-emulsification cataract surgery:

- Endophthalmitis (0.1%)
- Posterior capsular thickening (20%)
- Retinal detachment (0.7%)
- Raised intraocular pressure (no data)
- Cystoid macula oedema (no data)
- Unscheduled postoperative eye examinations

Unscheduled postoperative eye examinations

If for any reason you need to examine a patient's eye immediately after their surgery or prior to their planned follow-up or discharge visit, the following advice may be helpful. First, check the patient's notes. You need to see whether the operation was straightforward or whether there were any complications (e.g. posterior capsular tear, anterior vitrectomy and an anterior chamber lens was used instead of the usual posterior chamber lens). Ask the patient how they are feeling. Check their vision with and without a pinhole. Unless there were surgical complications, or the patient has developed an early inflammation or infection, vision should be slightly improved.

 Eyelid swelling: Unexpected eyelid swelling may indicate an allergy to eye-drops (or their preservatives) or an infection.

Poor vision

There are several reasons for poor vision in the intermediate postoperative period.

 Leaking wound: altering the refractive power of the cornea may cause the vision to be reduced. (Reduced vision is often referred to as 'vision is down'.)

 Corneal oedema: leads to reduced vision that does not improve with the use of a pinhole occluder (may be due to raised intraocular pressure, Fuchs' dystrophy, etc.).

 Perforation of the globe or optic nerve by local anaesthetic needle: exceedingly rare due to the increasing popularity of topical anaesthesia.

 Infection: postoperative endophthalmitis is an infection inside the eye that requires vitreous biopsy and intravitreal antibiotic treatment and is a danger to sight and to the eye's internal structures, even when treatment is started urgently (symptoms are pain and a rapid decrease in vision, but the intraocular pressure is normal).

 Intraocular lens error: it is incorrectly positioned or has the wrong prescription.

 Vitreous haemorrhage: particularly in people with diabetes.

 Monocular diplopia: caused by an intraocular lens (IOL) shifting position or folds in the posterior capsule or cystoid macula oedema.

 Soft lens matter: a small amount retained in the anterior chamber will clear naturally in time.

 Astigmatism: phaco-emulsification surgery and self-sealing wounds have reduced this problem and by careful evaluation of preoperative refraction, and considered location of their incisions, some surgeons are reducing preoperative astigmatisms (Ben Simon and Desatnik, 2004).

Problems with the wound

 Wound leak: may develop later in an eye that had a wound that was self-sealing at the end of the operation. Patients occasionally ring the hospital to complain of a sudden sharp pain and lacrimation followed by a reduction in vision. On examination they are seen to have an iris prolapse and possibly a shallow anterior chamber and low intraocular pressure. A leak can be confirmed by using Seidel's test (see Chapter 14 Basic Ophthalmic Procedures). Sometimes a prolapsed iris remains undetected until the follow-up clinic examination.

Problems with the cornea

 Corneal oedema: may occur following complicated surgery.

 Folds in Descemet's membrane: may occur following complicated surgery.

Problems with the anterior chamber

 Flat anterior chamber.

 Hyphaema.

 Hypopion.

Refractive problems

The intraocular lens may be poorly positioned, leading to poor vision. It may even be of the wrong prescription (this is referred to by the medical staff as a 'refractive surprise').

Problems inside the eye

 Vitreous prolapse: very rare and may follow complicated surgery that required an anterior vitrectomy.

 Uveitis/iritis: commonly occurs following intraocular surgery or eye injury. Patients are routinely prescribed steroid eye-drops post cataract surgery to control it. The inflammation is generally mild and normally clears in about two weeks.

Problems with the retina

 Loss of the red reflex: particularly relevant if the vision is 'down' as this is one of the observations the ophthalmologist will expect you to have made when you report the problem.

Problems with intraocular pressure

 Raised intraocular pressure: it is often raised a little in the first few hours following any intraocular surgery. If the operation was complicated, or the patient has glaucoma, the surgeon may prescribe acetazolamide to be taken in the immediate postoperative period, as raised intraocular pressure increases the risk of developing retinal vein occlusion, retinal artery occlusion or damage to their optic nerve. Evaluate raised intraocular pressure in relation to the preoperative intraocular pressure.

 Sudden, painful rise in intraocular pressure: this is always potentially serious.

Telephone advice

If the patient is more likely to develop one of the postoperative problems above, either as a result of a pre-existing eye condition or surgical complications, the surgeon may arrange to see them personally within the first postoperative week. Concerned patients or relatives may ring for advice prior to the nurse-led cataract outpatient appointment. The ophthalmic nurse is accountable for deciding whether to arrange to see the patient or to give telephone advice. The most frequently addressed problems are:

The patient worries that they are unable to see clearly enough to read. This is to be expected. The focus alters postoperatively as the new lens does not have the same focal range as the natural lens. Reading vision will be restored with new glasses.

The patient feels there is something in his or her eye, like a bit of grit or an eyelash. This is to be expected. The operation involved a series of puncture wounds that creates this sensation. It will settle in time.

The patient has a watery eye. Watering due to irritation around the incision is normal. Additionally, eye-drops given postoperatively may absorb moisture from the surface of the eye and create symptoms of dry eye.

The patient notices that their vision is becoming slowly worse since the operation.
 The patient needs to be seen as soon as possible back in the clinic. It could be caused by any of a number of simple problems, but occasionally it is a symptom of something more serious that requires treatment.

The patient wonders when he or she can drive again.
This will depend on the vision of the unoperated eye. The patient can do a SELF TEST by reading a number plate with both eyes at 62 feet (20.5 metres). If the patient makes a telephone query, and the patient's notes are not readily available we are not able to advise.

The patient wants advice about using postoperatively prescribed eye-drops.
Usually the treatment is four times a day and the course of treatment lasts for 4–6 weeks. During the postoperative follow-up visit, the drop dosage can be reviewed and decreased. Glaucoma treatment continues as before unless instructed differently by the surgeon. Pilocarpine eye-drops are the only ones that are routinely discontinued.

The postoperative review

In most eye units it is common for experienced nurses with expanded roles to examine the eye, to vary and reduce the eye-drop regimen, to list for the second eye or discharge patients. Exceptions to this may be combined surgeries (e.g. cataract and trabeculectomy) or the postoperative care of patients whose surgery was quite complicated. In many ophthalmic departments, nurses now manage all the routine postoperative reviews, but must develop sufficient confidence to ensure that ophthalmologists take responsibility for patients that lie outside the nursing remit.

At the postoperative review, the patient has an opportunity to ask any questions regarding their vision and hospital staff are able to determine and document the outcome of the surgery. The patient's distance vision is measured. This is done unaided, as the patient's current spectacles will no longer be the correct prescription for the operated eye. The postoperative spectacle prescription is also estimated, using an auto-refract machine.

There may be some problem establishing whether patients who wear spectacles see better with or without them. This may be because there is now a difference between the refractive power of the eyes of 3 dioptres or more. The brain cannot fuse the two differently sized pictures it perceives into one image. One spectacle lens may need to be temporarily covered in order to overcome this. The surgeon will need to know too, because it may be that the surgery on the patient's second eye will need to be brought forward.

Autorefract machine

This machine electronically generates a spectacle prescription by measuring the eye. The reading can be informative if the patient is not happy with the outcome of their vision. Often the vision can be improved by a slight spectacle prescription. Looking at the reading from the machine, the nurse can reassure the patient that their vision will improve once they have seen their optician (if the machine provides a simulated test). If a simulated vision test is not possible with the equipment provided, the nurse may need to put the required lenses into a trial frame and check that the patient's vision is adequate.

If the patient is very short-sighted, it is important to look at the biometry reading and the size of the implant used by the surgeon. This will enable the experienced nurse to work out the corrective prescription the surgeon was aiming for in terms of 'balancing' the two eyes to avoid the problems of anisometropia (see Chapter 3). This can then be compared with the reading from the auto-refract machine.

Problems may occur with auto-refraction if the machine is unable to record because:

- the patient's pupil is too small
- there are problems involving the cornea
- the·eye is amblyopic
- the patient is unable to focus their gaze into the machine
- the patient has head tremor.

Nursing examination of the postoperative cataract patient

Examine the patient's notes, then welcome the patient. Check the visual patient's acuity and auto-refract readings. Ask the patient how he or she has been feeling since the eye surgery while looking at their face for signs of personal stress, asymmetry or swelling of the eyelids. Carry out a full slit lamp examination of both eyes.

Table 7.1 gives a summary of possible problems that will require careful evaluation and consultation with the ophthalmologist. Generally eye-drop toxicity and eye-drop allergy may be managed with a nurse protocol.

Postoperative uveitis

Uveitis is often noticed at the postoperative visit, and usually settles with the help of postoperative steroid eye-drops. The inflammation may be more severe if the cataract surgery was complicated. Some patients have previous histories of bouts of uveitis and may need medical, rather than nursing, follow-up. Patients with severe postoperative iritis complain of blurred vision, photophobia and pain. Fibrin may be noted in the anterior chamber, and the patient will need to be seen by an ophthalmologist. Increased doses of steroid eye-drops, used over a slightly longer period, are necessary. Raised intraocular pressure may occur secondary to steroid use (if the patient is a 'steroid responder') or as a response to inflammation as above.

Postoperative visual problems

Cystoid macula oedema

Patients with this condition often complain of misty vision following surgery; the ophthalmologist – following pupil dilatation and a fundus check – diagnoses cystoid macula oedema. This relatively rare condition is more likely following complicated cataract surgery, or if the patient is diabetic. It typically occurs about 6–10 weeks after surgery (Kanski, 2007).

Endophthalmitis

This may manifest in two ways:

 As severe eye pain and reduced vision in the first week following surgery.

With delayed-onset from 4 weeks postoperatively (Kanski, 2007) in a slightly milder form. Cells and flare post surgery may fail to clear as expected and 'mutton fat' deposits may develop on the anterior surface of the cornea. There may be minor folds in Descemet's membrane and white plaque may develop on the posterior capsule.

Deposits forming on the intraocular lens implant

Fortunately, deposits forming on the intraocular lens implant are a rare occurrence. They can cause a decrease in vision and glare up to 10 years post surgery (Trevidi *et al.*, 2002). It is normal to remove and replace these lenses.

Capsular phimosis

This is caused by fibrosis and opacification of the capsulorhexis margin. Marked shrinkage of the

Table 7.1 *Postoperative examination conducted at the nurses' cataract clinic at Bournemouth Eye Unit*

Examination of	Observations	Possible problem
Lids	Sticky eyelashes	Infection
Conjunctiva	Redness Swelling	Infection or allergy 🚩
Cornea	Haziness	Oedema Raised IOP 🚩 Uveitis 🚩
	Punctate keratitis	Eye-drop or preservative allergy Dry eye
Pupil	Irregular	Sphincter rupture (? iris hooks or capsular tension ring used during surgery) Adhesions to capsule (uveitic eyes) 🚩 Vitreous in anterior chamber 🚩
	Peaked	Caught in wound 🚩
IOL	Check position	Should be clear (not tilted or displaced)
Anterior chamber	Depth (shallow)	Suggests wound leak 🚩
	Cells and flare	+ Usual + + Uveitis 🚩 + + + Possible hypopyon 🚩
	Fibrin	Denotes inflammation or infection 🚩
	Lens matter	Will absorb
Posterior chamber	Thickening or cloudiness of posterior capsule	Reduced vision May need laser
Wound	Leaking	Low IOP 🚩
Red reflex	If lost	Blood in vitreous 🚩 Pus in vitreous 🚩 Retinal detachment 🚩 Choroidal detachment 🚩
Vision	Lower than expected	Astigmatism Central macular oedema 🚩 Pre-existing AMD/POAG

AMD: age-related macular degeneration;

IOL: intraocular lens;

IOP: intraocular pressure;

POAG: primary open-angle glaucoma.

capsular margin leads to decreased vision. Dilating the pupil reveals the opaque, contracted anterior capsule opening that has led to the patient's decreased vision. Treatment is to enlarge the capsular opening using a YAG laser.

Posterior capsular fibrosis

This used to be a common post surgical problem. Decreased vision, photophobia and glare are possible symptoms of this now fairly rare problem that has been reduced by changing the design of intraocular lenses. Intraocular lenses with sharp rather than rounded edges are now the implants of choice (Findl *et al.*, 2007).

Silicone oil

Silicone oil may stick to the back of the IOL causing visual loss. Trevidi *et al.* (2002) state that silicone intraocular lenses are not recommended for patients who have had, or are likely to have, silicone oil inserted into their eye.

Retinal problems

Retinal problems such as detachments sometimes occur postoperatively. Often they are linked to difficult surgery with vitreous loss.

Discharge protocol

There is normally a single postoperative examination of the patient prior to re-listing for the second eye or discharge to the optometrist. Table 7.2 is provided as an example protocol for this responsibility. Utmost care needs to be taken with patients who have other eye pathology (e.g. glaucoma, retinal naevi) to ensure that they continue to be followed up in appropriate clinics.

At Bournemouth Eye Unit, only experienced nurses who have completed basic eye training, have worked under supervision and have consistently demonstrated all the in-house 'Competencies for Post Operative Examination' may discharge patients. They may only discharge patients following the surgeon's instructions in the patient's notes if:

- there is no other ophthalmic pathology
- if the visual acuity is 6/12 or better.

 Focus on Cataracts by the NHS Institute for Innovation and Improvement is a 'must read' to check whether your cataract service could be made even better.

Conclusions

The ophthalmic nurse's role in preoperative preparation, perioperative care, follow-up and postoperative discharge of cataract patients is key in providing expert care to this large group of patients. It requires good background nursing experience and the ability to manage patients who often have a range of other medical, mobility and domestic problems in their background. Outsiders may note the apparently restricted range of this role, but in fact it requires a comprehensive and deep knowledge of ophthalmic conditions that may coexist in the cataract patient's eye. There are also potential dangers that may arise because ophthalmic nurses are expected to settle quickly into this subspecialty before they have a chance to develop an adequate level of practical and theoretical knowledge.

Table 7.2 *Nursing discharge protocol (with permission from Bournemouth Eye Unit).*

	Follow-up	Discharge to optician	Same-day doctor advice/referral
Glaucoma	3–4 months	–	–
Age-related macular degeneration (AMD)	Wet AMD as consultant instructions	Yes	–
Diabetes with no retinopathy	–	Yes	–
Diabetes with retinopathy	As consultant instructions	–	–
Eyes look nice but visual acuity down ⚑	–	–	Yes
Retinal naevus (being observed)	As consultant instructions	–	–
Vitreous in anterior chamber ⚑	–	–	Yes ⚑
Floaters newly seen by patient	–	–	Yes ⚑
History of previous floaters (still seeing them)	–	Yes	Yes ⚑

References and further reading

Ben Simon, G. and Desatnik, H. (2004). Correction of pre-existing astigmatism during cataract surgery. *Graefe's Archive for Clinical and Experimental Ophthalmology* 243(4), 321–26.

Dinkaran, S., Desai, S. and Raj, P. (2000). Is the first postoperative day review necessary following uncomplicated phaco-emulsification surgery? *Eye*, 14(3a), 364–66.

Findl, O., Buehl, W., Bauer, P. and Sycha, T. (2007). Interventions for preventing posterior capsular opacification. *Cochrane Database of Systemic Reviews*. CD003738, 1469–93.

Kanski, J. (2007). *Clinical Ophthalmology. A Systemic Approach*. London: Butterworth Heinemann.

NHS Executive (2000). *Action on Cataracts: Good Practice Guidance*. London: NHS Executive.

NHS Institute for Innovation and Improvement (2007). *Focus On: Cataracts*. Coventry: NHS Institute.

Noble, B. and Simmons, I. (2001). *Complications of Cataract Surgery*. Oxford: Butterworth Heinemann.(An excellent book on the complications of cataract surgery for ophthalmologists that may be in your medical library. It is well worth browsing for deeper information.)

Tinley, C., Frost, A., Hakin, K., McDermott, W. and Ewings, P. (2003). Is visual outcome compromised when next day review is omitted after phaco-emulsification surgery? A randomised controlled trial. *British Journal of Ophthalmology*, 87(11), 1350–55.

Trevidi, R., Werner, L., Apple, D., Pandey, S. and Izak, A. (2002). Post cataract intraocular lens (IOP) surgery opacification. *Eye*, 16, 217–41.

Useful web resources

NHS Institute for Innovation and Improvement: Focus on Cataracts
http://www.institute.nhs.uk/
How to make cataract services even better.

Good Hope Hospital
http://www.goodhope.org.uk/
Check this site for the glaucoma progression model, glaucoma progression text and trabeculectomy animation.

Medrounds
http://www.medrounds.org/
Check for useful articles and video clips of surgery.

Royal College of Ophthalmologists
http://www.rcophth.ac.uk/docs/publications/CataractSurgeryGuidelinesMarch2005Updated.pdf
Provides guidelines on a wide range of matters around cataract surgery, such as use of local anaesthetic, warfarin and aspirin and cataract surgery, issues around biometry, choice of intraocular lens, epidemiology and cataract outcomes.

SELF TEST answers on page 205

1. Give two 'red flag' symptoms that might occur in the first 24 hours following surgery.

2. In 1999 the Department of Health identified posterior capsular thickening as a complication that affects 20% of postoperative cataract patients. Why might this data be incorrect now?

3. Why is endophthalmitis very serious?

4. Postoperative measurement of a patient's visual acuity should be done without spectacles. Why?

5. If there is a difference of 3 dioptres or more between a patient's eyes postoperatively, what visual symptom is the patient likely to complain of? How is this problem managed?

6. Why might a patient have unusually severe uveitis in the postoperative period?

_____

_____

_____

7. Give two possible reasons for raised intraocular pressure in a patient attending a cataract follow-up/discharge clinic.

_____

_____

_____

_____

Chapter 8

The glaucomas, primary open-angle glaucoma and congenital glaucoma

Lynn Ring

Glaucoma seems to be a very confusing subject at first, until you realise that it is not a single disorder but a wide range of disorders grouped together under one collective name. One way of appreciating the range of disorders covered by glaucoma is to think about chest disease. Many chest diseases cause breathlessness, but a list of those diseases might include cancer of the lung, acute bronchitis, chronic obstructive airways disease and asthma – it is immediately obvious that they have different causes, a wide range of lung changes and diverse treatment options. Similarly, glaucoma is the name given to a large group of eye conditions that eventually leads to damage at the optic nerve head (or optic disc as it is otherwise known).

The glaucomas are divided into primary glaucomas and secondary glaucomas. This chapter and the two that follow present reasonably deep information about the dynamics of glaucoma, the variety of conditions within the broad classification of primary and secondary glaucoma, and how nurses can help patients to care for themselves at home. This will help new nurses in particular to provide attention with the patient as the focus. It is necessary to appreciate that in the UK 2 % of people over the age of 40 and 10 % of the people aged over 70 have this condition, and that 25 % of NHS hospital eye service outpatient appointments are for primary open-angle glaucoma and ocular hypertension (National Institute for Health and Clinical Excellence, 2007). A significant number of ophthalmic nurses are developing advanced prescribing roles within this area of clinical practice and at an early stage of development will be expected to develop the skill of Goldman applanation tonometry.

Intraocular pressure (IOP) will be discussed in addition to how it affects sight by impacting on the nerve fibre layer within the retina. It is anticipated that the information presented will stimulate further reading and exploration of this fascinating subject. New nurses are particularly encouraged to discuss their newly acquired knowledge with senior nurses and medical staff to further integrate this knowledge into their everyday practice. Internet sites are referenced for theatre nurses to describe surgery through the use of diagrams and video clips.

Intraocular pressure

The eye requires a certain level of intraocular pressure to function naturally. This pressure is dependent on a continuous process of aqueous formation and drainage. Aqueous is produced by the radial ciliary processes of the ciliary body. Active secretion of the aqueous is a metabolic process relying on the sodium–potassium pump secreting ions into the posterior chamber. The normal intraocular pressure of the eye, varying from 10–21 mmHg per individual, is maintained by an equilibrium between the rate of aqueous formation and its outflow via the trabecular meshwork. There is a natural diurnal curve to intraocular pressure readings, usually being higher in the mornings and reducing over the rest of the day.

To do ...

Look at the diagram of the eye in Fig. 2.1 (p.7). Identify the ciliary body and the canal of Schlemm. Visualise the passage of aqueous from the posterior chamber into the drainage angle (as illustrated in Fig. 2.7, p.16).

The uveoscleral pathway

Aqueous exits the eye via the **trabecular pathway** (sometimes called 'the conventional route') which accounts for approximately 90% of aqueous outflow (Kanski, 2007). The cells of the trabecular meshwork act as a pressure-sensitive system to allow aqueous into the canal of Schlemm, and then to the episcleral veins, which are drained by the venous circulation. However, more recently greater attention has been focused on the **uveoscleral pathway** that accounts for approximately 10% of aqueous outflow (Snell and Lemp, 1998). Gabelt and Kaufman (1978) describe how (at normal intraocular pressure) aqueous slowly seeps through the face of the ciliary body just posterior to the scleral spur in the apex of the anterior chamber angle. As there are no epithelial, endothelial or dense connective tissue-filled spaces between the ciliary muscle bundles, the anterior chamber is, in effect, continuous with those spaces. The inter-muscle connective tissue, while providing some resistance to the flow, is sufficiently porous to allow fluid movement into the supraciliary and suprachoroidal spaces, and from there to leak through the sclera wall into the surrounding periocular orbital tissues. This flow is constant, independent of intraocular pressure in normal eyes. Research interest in the uveoscleral outflow route has grown in recent years with the discovery that prostaglandin substances, and analogues such as latanoprost (Xalatan™) lower intraocular pressure by increasing the uveoscleral drainage. This has led to the development of new treatment strategies for glaucoma.

Tonometry

Measuring the intraocular pressure is a key feature of an eye examination. Goldman applanation tonometry is used in hospitals to measure intraocular pressure in adults. You can read more about how these readings are obtained in Chapter 14 on basic ophthalmic procedures. The prism may be single-use only and to be disposed of appropriately, or re-usable and to be sterilised between patients.

The primary glaucomas include:

- primary infantile glaucoma

- primary open-angle glaucoma
- primary closed-angle glaucoma.

Primary infantile glaucoma

This form of glaucoma is fortunately very rare, but the potential effects on the child's general development can be very disabling. Early recognition, appropriate treatment and continued monitoring can significantly improve the child's visual outcome and early personal development. All infantile glaucomas arise from developmental anomalies of the trabecular meshwork, leading to increased intraocular pressure and resulting in loss of vision. Kanski (2007) classifies them as:

- congenital (40%) – exists in utero
- infantile (55%) – manifest by age 3
- juvenile (5%) – manifest by age 16.

Generally a child with primary infantile glaucoma has a history of at least two relatives with glaucoma. The symptoms of primary infantile glaucoma are likely to involve:

- a hazy cornea
- epiphora (excessive tearing)
- photophobia
- blepharospasm (spasm or squeezing of the eyelids).

Any child with these symptoms should have a full examination under an anaesthetic which would include tonometry using a hand-held tonometer (the 'Perkins' is generally used) and measurement of the corneal diameter. A corneal diameter of greater than 12 mm before the child is 1 year old is a strong indicator for primary infantile glaucoma. If left untreated, the child's eyes (Cibis *et al.* 2006 say that in 75% of children, both eyes are affected) become larger because the cornea and sclera in the very young stretch readily and become swollen and engorged. Male children are the most frequently affected, accounting for 65% of all cases (Cibis *et al.*, 2006).

Treatment options are almost always surgical intervention. Ocular hypotensive drugs may be used to reduce the intraocular pressure in the interim but surgery has the greatest chance of preserving vision. The two most common surgical procedures are goniotomy and trabeculectomy. Both procedures involve incisions to increase aqueous drainage via the trabecular meshwork. In goniotomy some of the trabecular meshwork fibres are cut to allow aqueous to flow more readily into the canal of Schlemm. In trabeculectomy, an alternative drainage route is created.

As infantile glaucoma is relatively rare, an expert paediatric ophthalmologist in a regional centre would usually treat it. Treatment 'success' will depend on the type of infantile glaucoma, the presence of other complications such as cataract and micro-cornea, and the criteria used to judge 'success'. Modern treatment results are encouraging (Biglan, 2006), but the child will require lifetime follow-up and generally supplementary treatments in terms of eye-drops are required.

To do ...

Find out if infantile glaucoma is treated within your own eye unit or referred on to a regional centre. Where is the regional centre? Does your eye unit have travel information available for the parents (as practicalities need to be considered at this stressful time)?

Primary open-angle glaucoma

Primary open-angle glaucoma (POAG) may be defined as being a group of conditions characterised by optic disc cupping and visual field loss caused by compression of the optic nerve fibres. The intraocular pressure may be moderately raised, or even high, although it is not always raised above the usual range of 10–21 mmHg. POAG predominantly affects the population over 40 years old (Kanski, 2007), but prevalence increases with age. It has a subtle, painless onset and generally affects both eyes although only one eye may be affected at diagnosis. Within the community, early detection by an optometrist can prevent sight loss from this and other eye disorders, therefore it is essential to encourage the general public (particularly those aged over 40) to attend regularly every 2 years for sight checks. The optometrist will check the intraocular pressure, optic disc and test the visual field.

There is no other ocular disease associated with POAG, therefore it is the primary problem. It is the most common of all the glaucomas and there may be a family history. It is responsible for approximately 12% of blind registrations in the UK and USA and remains the leading cause of blindness in African–Americans whereas it is the third leading cause amongst white people in the USA (Girkin, 2004).

THINK

What might be the factors underlying the reluctance of some people to visit their optometrist regularly?

Why might people who are entitled to a free sight test in the UK still be reluctant to attend?

POAG is the thief of sight; everyone is vulnerable to it. This is because in the early development of the problem, there are no obvious symptoms. The area of sharpest vision at the macula is not affected until very late in the disease. The progressive visual field loss is not evident to the patient until the condition reaches advanced stages. Typically the person develops an arcuate scotoma (an arc-shaped blind spot) in the upper nasal field of one eye, which slowly enlarges. This lack of initial awareness of anything being wrong is because the visual fields of both eyes overlap, and as one eye is likely to have more rapid visual field loss than the other, the second eye 'compensates' for a while. If the disease is left untreated, much larger blind spots develop and the person may eventually become effectively blind. This is why regular eye tests are essential to early diagnosis and treatment.

It is appropriate to mention here that very often people with advanced POAG are misunderstood in terms of their sight loss. They may still be capable of reading a book, because the macula may still be functional, but may easily become lost in unfamiliar surroundings because their constricted visual field will make it difficult for them to find their way. You should offer your assistance readily in the eye clinic; if you call a patient, make sure that they have seen you and are able to follow you. Offer an arm if necessary. Patients may still meet the eyesight requirements for driving in good daylight conditions but may find it very difficult to see anything much in twilight, even when walking about reasonably slowly. Try to keep the clinic environment well lit, and be prepared to help as necessary in dimly lit examination rooms.

Predisposing factors for POAG

Age: With an increasingly ageing population worldwide, it is estimated that over 4.5 million people will be bilaterally blind from primary open-angle glaucoma in 2010 (Quigley and Broman, 2006).

Ethnicity: Writing about a US population, Racette *et al.* (2003) estimated glaucoma to be six times more common in black people than white people, presenting 10 years earlier and progressing more rapidly. They question whether intraocular pressure may be underestimated in black people, who tend to have thinner corneas. Mercieca *et al.* (2007) showed that central corneal thickness was lower in various sub-Saharan, African–American and Afro–Caribbean groups than in white populations. The suggestion that patients with glaucoma are more likely to have a thinner cornea compared with a group of non-glaucomatous controls demonstrated a difference that was not statistically significant.

Genetics: POAG is often associated with a positive family history. Everyone with a positive family history, particularly involving a first-degree relative (i.e. a parent or sibling) should undergo an annual intraocular pressure, optic disc and visual field check at the optometrist's practice. The Nottingham Eye Study (Sung *et al.*, 2006) demonstrated that siblings of parents with POAG have an increased risk of developing it themselves, and that risk increases with age. Glaucoma patients should be encouraged to suggest that their family members are regularly screened. However, not everyone with a relative suffering from glaucoma will develop the disease themselves.

Myopia: Moderate and severe myopia are factors that increase the risk of developing open-angle glaucoma, although the direct mechanism is unknown (Loyo Berios and Blustein, 2007).

POAG is associated with several systemic disorders:

Diabetes: Many studies have questioned a possible relationship between diabetes and glaucoma. A study by de Voogd *et al.* (2006) concluded that diabetes was not a risk for open-angle glaucoma, but Pasquale *et al.* (2006) found type 2 diabetes was positively associated with open-angle glaucoma. Previously, Ellis *et al.* (2000) discussed the division of opinion on the potential association of diabetes with open-angle glaucoma and expressed their opinion that a detection bias has contributed to the association between diabetes and open-angle glaucoma.

Poor blood supply to the optic nerve: In addition to the significance of raised intraocular pressure leading to glaucomatous damage at the optic disc, a poor blood supply to the optic nerve is a recognised cause of damage to the optic disc and nerve fibres. Systemic hypotension and resultant poor diastolic perfusion is one of the major causative factors. Also implicated are migraine headaches and peripheral vascular spasm (American Academy of Ophthalmology, 2005).

Thyroid problems and glaucoma: Research by Cross *et al.* (2008) has lent support to the hypothesis that thyroid disorders may increase the risk of glaucoma. Studies are ongoing.

Developing POAG is generally linked with the predisposing factors above, but the exact mechanisms remain unknown. Patients with high intraocular pressures on presentation are more likely to develop progressive disease. The normal range for intraocular pressure is considered to be between 10 and 21 mmHg, however there are factors that potentially distort intraocular pressure readings, and the relative thickness or thinness of the central cornea will alter readings slightly. This is because the Goldman applanation technique assumes a central corneal thickness of 555 μm. Many eye units now measure corneal thickness using corneal pachymetry to identify potential variables in intraocular pressure readings.

Find out if your department measures central corneal thickness and how this is done.

Diagnosis of POAG

Early identification of people with POAG is critical to preservation of reasonable eyesight throughout their life. Patients are generally referred to the eye clinic because the community optometrist has found something unusual or abnormal after assessment of their intraocular pressure, optic disc and visual fields. A firm diagnosis of POAG depends on abnormalities being found in two out of three of these elements.

Optic disc assessment

Changes to the optic disc and the cup to disc ratio (CDR) may be reported by the optometrist following routine screening or noted by the ophthalmologist within the hospital eye service. Various instruments can be used to view the optic disc – the direct ophthalmoscope or the slit lamp, with additional non-contact lenses. A normal optic disc has certain features and a specific cup-to-disc thickness ratio. The thickest part of the neural retinal rim (NRR) should be the inferior segment. It should become gradually thinner superiorly and nasally reachingits thinnest temporally. Nurses learning to examine the optic disc often use the ISNT rule to check the four areas.

ISNT rule for checking the optic disk

I Inferior – thickest (where most nerve fibres pass from the optic nerve to the neural layer of the retina)

S Superior – thinner

N Nasal – thinner still

T Temporal – thinnest

There is an illustrated explanation of the cup to disc ratio by Kwon at the *Med Rounds* website. When you begin to learn to look at the optic disc, check out Bourne (2006).

Changes at the optic disc are difficult to evaluate without extensive experience in practice, as each person's discs have a slightly different appearance. Highly myopic people often have large optic discs with a greater cup to disc ratio and hypermetropic eyes have smaller optic discs. When a patient presents with an asymmetrical disc appearance, it should be a cause for concern. Similarly, the discovery of defects in the visual fields is a major concern.

Visual field assessment

Highly sensitive computer-controlled machines such as the Humphrey Field Analyzer™ are used to test the field of vision. The peripheral visual field is usually the first place where damage to the eyesight is evident. Approximately 20–40% of nerve fibre has to be damaged before visual loss is detectable.

Visual field testing is not always accurate as 'artefacts' may appear on the visual field print record, caused by something such as the edge of a patient's spectacle frame, or a drooping eyelid partially obscuring the pupil. Provision should be made for patients who are presbyopic to wear their reading spectacles for the test, or their distance spectacles should be measured on the focimeter and a calculation made for the reading lens which should be mounted on the fields machine prior to commencing the test.

Visual field testing is intimidating to patients; some have described the experience as being 'like putting your head inside an electric colander'. It can be very tiring for a stressed person and some people worry in case they 'get it wrong'; because of the stress, some people miss some of the more subtle target lights, making it look as if they have field defects. This is why visual field testing needs to be undertaken by a skilled technician and reviewed by an experienced ophthalmologist or ophthalmic nurse.

To do ...

Ask your fields technician to test your visual field so that you may experience how difficult it can be to obtain an accurate record for an older person on first testing.

THINK

From reading the above plus your conversations with the field technician, list the factors that must be borne in mind in order to obtain an accurate field test.

Listen to what patients have to say about their experience of visual field testing.

How might the nurse or technician improve their experience?

Discuss your answers with your mentor.

Normal tension glaucoma (NTG)

Some patients may present with normal intraocular pressure readings but have optic nerve damage and related loss in their visual fields. This is referred to as normal tension glaucoma (NTG) or normal pressure glaucoma (NPG). The optic disc may show focal damage in one area and splinter haemorrhages. The visual field defects tend to be deeper, producing more central visual symptoms. Central corneal thickness (CCT) may be a factor in this condition as the intraocular pressure reading could be a false low in a patient with a very thin cornea, and the patient's condition may not be noticed until field defects develop. Even though their intraocular pressure is normal, ophthalmologists treat NTG with eye-drops because a reduction in intraocular pressure by around 30 % has been shown to be beneficial in protecting the visual field (Hoyng and Kitazana, 2002).

Ocular hypertension (OHT)

Conversely, not all patients with raised intraocular pressure will present with either optic disc damage or visual field loss. This is referred to as ocular hypertension. It is here that central corneal thickness may play a part in diagnosis and treatment decisions. Raised intraocular pressure is a risk factor in developing optic disc damage and visual loss, but central corneal thickness may lead to false high readings.

To do ...

Ask the glaucoma consultant what factors are involved in making a decision to treat patients who only have raised intraocular pressure without concurrent disc and field damage.

THINK

Can it be safely assumed that 'suspect' glaucoma patients will attend for annual check ups with their community optometrist?

Medical treatments for primary open-angle glaucoma

Treatments may vary slightly between different eye units and the population being served. Generally, medical intervention (use of eye-drops) would be first-line treatment. A range of eye-drops is available to reduce intraocular pressures; they are selected by ophthalmologists on the basis of best available treatment and available funding. Noecker *et al.* (2007) state that 'fixed combination medications (monotherapy) offer the potential of maximising patient adherence by decreasing the burden of using multiple topical agents ... and by potentially decreasing the costs for the patient and the healthcare system' (see Table 8.1).

Compliance, concordance, adherence or persistence?

All these words have been used to discuss means of persuading patients to use their eye-drops regularly and at the prescribed time intervals. Compliance is often a word used in ophthalmic clinics. This implies that the patient does as he is told without knowledge or understanding of the rationale behind the prescription. Adherence to the prescription is the aim of any regimen, as taking the eye-drops means the intraocular pressure will become lower and the progressive nature of the disease will be slowed.

The most important thing to remember is that the best or even the most expensive of all the eye-drops available will not work if the patient fails to understand the importance of using them. Self-reporting of compliance by patients may be unreliable given that the amount of returned medications in the UK can be measured in many tons. It is known, however, that daily doses of medication are more likely to be taken (Benner, 2002). It is important that ophthalmologists involve their patients in treatment choices, by discussing available alternatives and potential side effects with them. Glaucoma clinics are notoriously busy and over-booked, often leaving the ophthalmologist with little time to fully investigate compliance issues. Nurses also know that patients often talk with them about matters they feel are too trivial to discuss with their doctor, because they do not want to bother the ophthalmologist, or they think their concerns are not important. Take the time to ask the patient if they are having any problems with their medications.

Table 8.1 *Glaucoma drugs*

Drug group	Contraindications	Side effects	
		Ocular	Systemic
BETA-BLOCKERS Timolol Metipranolol Levobunolol (Betagan™) Carteolol (Teoptic™) Betaxolol (Betoptic™)	Asthma COPD Bradycardia > 60 b.p.m. Heart block Cardiac failure	Rare: Epithelial keratopathy Reduced corneal sensation	Bradycardia Arrhythmia Heart failure Bronchospasm Depression Masked hypoglycaemia
PROSTAGLANDIN ANALOGUES Latanoprost (Xalatan™) Travoprost (Travatan™) Bimatoprost (Lumigan™) Xalacom™(combined timolol and Xalatan™) PROSTAGLANDINS + BETA-BLOCKER G Xalacom™ (timolol + Xalatan™) G Duo-Trav™ (timolol + Travatan™) G. Ganfort™ (timolol + Lumigan[tm])	None known (other than known hypersensitivity or allergy)	Increased iris pigmentation Increased lash length and thickness Increased eyelid pigmentation	Caution in severe asthma
CARBONIC ANHYDRASE INHIBITORS Dorzolamide (Trusopt™) Brinzolamide (Azopt™) Cosopt™ (dorzolamide + timolol) Acetazolamide oral medication CARBONIC ANHYDRASE INHIBITORS + BETA-BLOCKER G Cosopt™ (dorzolamide + timolol)	Severe kidney or liver disease if low sodium or potassium levels Allergy	Discomfort Discharge Blurred vision Itching	Metallic taste Dry mouth Fatigue Dyspnoea Headache Common side effects: nausea, vomiting, taste disturbance, headache, flushing, thirst, polyuria
NON-SELECTIVE SYMPATHOMIMETICS SELECTIVE SYMPATHOMIMETICS Apraclonidine (Iopidine™) Brimonidine (Alphagan P™) SELECTIVE SYMPATHOMIMETICS + BETA-BLOCKER G Combigan™ (brimonidine + timolol) Combigan™ (Alphagan™ + timolol)	MAOIs Tricyclic antidepressants Occludable angles Alphagan may have additive effect with CNS depressants Hypersensitivity	Tearing Hyperaemia Stinging Oedema	Dry mouth Fatigue Headache Bradycardia Depression
PARASYMPATHOMIMETICS Pilocarpine	Soft contact lens wearers Conditions where iris constriction is not advised (e.g. acute uveitis) Hypersensitivity	Miosis Accommodation spasm	(Extremely rare) Hypotension Bradycardia Bronchial spasm Pulmonary oedema Nausea and vomiting Sweating Diarrhoea

CNS: central nervous system;

COPD: chronic obstructive pulmonary disease;

MAOI: monoamine oxidase inhibitors.

References: British National Formulary (2006); Bartlett (2006); Salmon and Kanski (2004).

The overall aim of any ocular hypotensive therapy is to reduce the intraocular pressure and maintain useful sight. The difficulty is that sight loss in primary open-angle glaucoma is slow, insidious and undetectable until many nerve fibres have been lost. One of the main difficulties is to convince the patient that they need to follow the ophthalmologist's advice and take this eye-drop that can be uncomfortable, irritating and a general nuisance.

THINK

How many times have you been given antibiotics for an infection and told to complete the course, but felt better and then missed the last few doses because you forgot?

Think how much more difficult it would have been if you had not been feeling unwell in the first place.

How significant might prescription costs be to a working person with a family?

POAG is asymptomatic. It is difficult for the patient to believe that their eyesight may deteriorate when they have no existing difficulties. Communication is a vital component of the relationship between the ophthalmologist and patient. But how long is the appointment for – only 10 or 15 minutes? This is why the nurse is uniquely placed to offer advice and support to a patient who does not really understand why the drops matter.

However, compliance implies that the patient is a passive recipient of the ophthalmologist's orders to adhere to their regimen. Remember all those forgotten antibiotics! Should the patient be the passive partner or should there be an equal partnership between the ophthalmologist and patient? Should there be an implicit understanding between two equals of the responsibilities that lie with each partner? These questions are posed deliberately.

Phasing tests

Even the most compliant, adherent patient may continue to develop visual field changes. It is for these patients that the nurse may be asked to arrange a phasing test. Phasing is where a patient attends the eye unit all day and has an intraocular pressure check every hour. The nurse is often responsible for these investigations and the results show the ophthalmologist how the patient is responding to eye-drops across the natural diurnal fluctuation of intraocular pressure. Imagine that the intraocular pressure was always checked at much the same time during an afternoon clinic. The diurnal peak morning pressure would be missed due to the time of day the intraocular pressure was checked.

If medical intervention is unable to achieve a drop in intraocular pressure to prevent progressive vision loss there are other treatment options. Laser and surgery would both be considered. However, as there are risks with all interventions, the ophthalmologist will need to ensure that the patient is aware of the options and the risk–benefit continuum as part of the consent to treatment process.

 Progression models for glaucoma may be seen at the **Good Hope Hospital** website.

Laser treatments

Laser trabeculoplasty (LTP)

Laser trabeculoplasty is a technique that uses an argon laser to treat open-angle glaucoma. Using a specialised contact lens applied to the cornea, the laser beam is accurately focused to deliver a precise burst of light energy that burns tiny holes through the trabecular meshwork. As these areas heal, subsequent contraction around the burn sites 'pulls' or 'stretches' these microscopic channels further open, increasing drainage of fluid into the canal of Schlemm and decreasing the intraocular pressure.

Selective laser trabeculoplasty (SLT)

Selective laser trabeculoplasty is a newer, non-thermal laser technology that uses an Nd:YAG laser to irradiate only the melonin-rich cells within the trabecular meshwork, thus causing less damage to the surrounding cells. Theoretically this means that further treatment should be possible if the effects of the original treatment are inadequate. However the results of long-term clinical trials are awaited.

Nursing care of the patient requiring laser trabeculoplasty

All nursing staff need to be aware that this treatment is aimed at reducing the intraocular pressure. It will not improve the patient's eyesight, but will help to preserve what is left.

The patient requires instillation of miotic (pupil-constricting) eye-drops, usually pilocarpine, which may produce a headache or brow-ache and cause blurred vision. The nurse will need to ensure that the patient knows about the anticipated side effects of these drops. The procedure takes approximately 5 minutes and is performed on the appropriate laser machine, which looks similar to a slit lamp. Patients are often very anxious prior to laser treatment and the nurse can offer reassurance and support during this time. Laser treatment tends to be painless but can sometimes feel like pinpricks, so discuss this with the patient.

During the treatment a caution light ('Laser treatment – Do not enter') must be displayed outside the closed door of the room. If a nurse needs to stay with the patient, perhaps to help them keep their head in the correct position or if they are particularly nervous, then the correct goggles must be worn for the duration of the treatment.

After the treatment, the patient must wait for 1 hour for a check of intraocular pressure. This is because there may be a critical rise in the intraocular pressure immediately post treatment, which is highly undesirable for patients whose vision is already compromised by chronically raised pressure.

Any elevation in pressure from the pre-treatment level must be reported to the ophthalmologist immediately. Apraclonidine may be routinely prescribed as a statutory dose immediately post treatment to prevent this, but the post-treatment check is essential. Oral acetazolamide (Diamox) is occasionally required to control the intraocular pressure on discharge.

Patients are discharged on anti-inflammatory drops used four times daily for 1 week to reduce the inflammation caused by the laser treatment. Often only a section of the drainage angle is lasered at each visit, which means that patients may need repeated treatments to achieve the greatest lowering effect on intraocular pressure. Patients must always continue their ocular hypotensive drops unless directed otherwise. If laser treatment is unsuccessful, then glaucoma surgery may be required.

Trabeculectomy

Preoperative preparation and nursing care

At the initial interview counsel the patient regarding the appropriate preoperative preparation for this surgery. It is often performed under local anaesthetic but may be offered under general anaesthetic, so the patient needs to know if a period of fasting is required. Check the surgeon's wishes regarding whether the patient should instil or omit their regular topical or systemic ocular hypotensive medication on the day of surgery. They may be instructed to omit them to increase the amount of aqueous flowing through the newly formed bleb. Often patients do not remember everything that is told to them, so they should be given a printed leaflet about the procedure to support the verbal information they are given.

On arrival, preparations for local or general anaesthesia will need to be made. The pupil should be miosed with eye-drops according to the local protocol to facilitate the peripheral iridectomy that will be an intrinsic part of the trabeculectomy procedure. The consent form will need to be checked.

Intraoperative procedure

The goal of this surgery is to lower the intraocular pressure by creating a surgical channel that allows aqueous to flow out from the anterior chamber and bubble up under the conjunctiva. From there it will be absorbed by the conjunctival blood vessels. You will need to carefully study the surgical approaches, which differ slightly from surgeon to surgeon.

 You can see a really helpful animated illustration of what the surgeon is doing stage by stage at the Good Hope Hospital website.

An initial 'bridle' suture may be inserted into the cornea to steady the eye during surgery. Then the operation site is positioned superiorly so that the upper eyelid protects it. A conjunctival flap is constructed. Many surgeons use antimetabolite drugs to stop failure of the operation by preventing the scleral flap from healing closed. The sclera is treated with sponges soaked in mitomycin C (0.5–0.2 mg/mL) or 5-fluorouracil (50 mg/mL) at this stage, without touching the conjunctiva. The animation can be found at the Good Hope Hospital website.

An initial partial-thickness flap of sclera is cut (the surgeon may have indicated the area of the proposed flap first, using tiny cautery marks or a dye). This scleral flap is dissected back as far as the cornea. A tiny block of full-thickness sclera is excised.

The peripheral iris is secured with forceps and iris scissors are used to cut a triangular-shaped peripheral iridectomy. The initial scleral flap is carefully folded back like a 'trapdoor' and loosely tacked back at the corners (some surgeons use adjustable sutures that in the postoperative period are used to titrate the amount of fluid draining from the anterior chamber). Then the conjunctiva is sutured.

Some surgeons like to inject a little balanced salt solution into the eye to raise the bleb. This looks like a 'blister' on the conjunctiva. The conjunctival blood vessels collect and drain aqueous from this area. Atropine 1% or homatropine 1% eye-drops may be instilled at the end of the procedure to dilate the pupil slightly and reduce the rate of drainage initially from the eye.

 There are surgical videos that you can watch at the AOL video website.

Postoperative care

To improve the flow of aqueous through the bleb, the surgeon usually discontinues glaucoma medications. Topical medications for the prevention of infection and inflammation consisting of antibiotic drops four times a day and anti-inflammatory drops (e.g. prednisolone drops 2-hourly are prescribed). A cartella shield is applied to cover the eye until the following morning when it can be removed. It should then be washed and kept clean for use only at night.

 Warn patients that any pain should be controlled with over-the-counter analgesia such as paracetamol or ibuprofen. If at any stage the pain becomes uncontrolled or their vision decreases, the patient should be asked to contact the eye unit immediately or at night they should contact the local eye accident and emergency department. The postoperative period for trabeculectomy is likely to involve many visits to the outpatient department, and patients need to be prepared for this. The postoperative period may include interventions such as:

● massage of the drainage bleb to increase the flow of aqueous into the bleb

● laser suture lysis to increase aqueous flow

● loosening of adjustable flap sutures with forceps at the slit lamp

● further antimetabolite drugs.

Complications of trabeculectomy surgery

Normally the bleb can be viewed when the upper lid is lifted. The bleb may fail if it is not formed in the first few postoperative days. Bleb leakage may cause a flat bleb.

A flat or shallow anterior chamber may develop due to over-drainage. This must be re-formed to prevent corneal decompensation. Indeed, hypotony (an intraocular pressure below 5 mmHg) will also require wound revision. Choroidal detachment may occur as a result of very low intraocular pressure.

Suprachoroidal haemorrhage may occur due to rupture of the long posterior ciliary artery as a result of progressive stretching with increasing serous choroidal detachment. This fortunately very rare complication may occur several days after trabeculectomy, and presents initially with sudden intense eye pain and visual loss.

There is increased prevalence of cataract formation. Many ophthalmologists will, in recognition of this, combine trabeculectomy with cataract surgery.

To do ...

Ask an ophthalmologist in the glaucoma clinic to show you what a filtration bleb looks like.

Glaucoma filtration valve implants

There are a variety of these devices on the market. They are used to treat patients with a poor surgical prognosis, such as those with previously failed trabeculectomy surgery, a complicated eye condition or previous eye surgery. The Ahmed™ glaucoma valve is reasonably popular at time of writing. Theatre nurses may care to watch videos that show how the surgeon fits this valve and other named valves. See the suggestions at the end of this chapter.

Complications of filtration valve surgery

These include hyphaema, gradual exposure of the valve plate, blockage of the tube and hypotony.

Postoperative care

For patients undergoing filtration valve implantation, postoperative care is similar to that provided for trabeculectomy.

Conclusions

From your work in the eye unit you will probably have noticed that dealing with POAG is a major part of the everyday workload of every department, because it may be a patient's primary eye condition or it may co-exist with another eye condition. This means that all staff should be vigilant to ensure that patients who have had, for example, cataract or eyelid surgery are not discharged until someone has checked they have a follow-up appointment for their glaucoma, that they understand what they must do regarding their glaucoma medications, and that they have an adequate supply of these medications.

The Royal College of Ophthalmologists (2009) estimated that 25% of all follow-up patients and 15% of all new referrals are either glaucoma patients or suspected of having glaucoma. This was a crippling load to be borne by the medical staff, and with consultant ophthalmologist support, ophthalmic nurses have expanded their roles over recent years to include optic disc assessment, Goldman tonometry, visual field testing and interpretation and patient advice and support. Increasing numbers of nurses are taking on nurse prescribing responsibilities and additional training and education to specialise within the field of glaucoma and are running clinics as a valued part of the glaucoma service in their area.

References and further reading

American Academy of Ophthalmology (2005). *Preferred practice patterns. Primary open-angle glaucoma.* San Francisco: The Eye MD Association.

Bartlett, J.D. (2006). *Ophthalmic Drug Facts.* St Louis: Wolters Kluwer.

Benner, J., Glynn, R., Mogun, H., *et al.* (2002). Long-term persistence in the use of statin therapy in elderly patients. *Journal of the American Medical Association*, **288**(4), 455–61.

Biglan, A. (2006). Glaucoma in children: Are we making progress? *Journal of American Association for Pediatric Ophthalmology and Strabismus*, **10**(1), 7–21.

Bourne, R. (2006). The optic nerve head in glaucoma. *Community Eye Health*, **19**(59), 44–45.

British National Formulary (2006). *British National Formulary 2006.* Biggleswade: BMJ Publishing Group Ltd and Royal Pharmaceutical Society of Great Britain.

Cibis, G., Urban, R. and Choplin, M. (2006). Glaucoma, primary congenital.
Available at: http://www.emedicine.com/oph/topic138.htm (last accessed August 2009).

Cross, J., Girkin, C., Owsley, C. and McGwin, G. (2008). The association between thyroid problems and glaucoma. *British Journal of Ophthalmology*, **92**(11), 1503–05.

de Voogd, S., Ikram, M., Wolfs, R., *et al.* (2006). Is diabetes mellitus a risk factor for open-angle glaucoma? The Rotterdam Study. *Ophthalmology*, **113**(10), 1827–31.

Ellis, J., Evans, J., Ruta, D., *et al.* (2000). Glaucoma incidence in an unselected cohort of diabetic patients: Is diabetes mellitus a risk factor for glaucoma? *British Journal of Ophthalmology*, **84**(11), 1218–24.

Gabelt, B. and Kaufman, P. (1978). Uveoscleral outflow. Biology and clinical aspects. In: A. Alm, P. Kaufman, Y. Kitazawa, *et al. Uveoscleral Outflow. Biology and Clinical Aspects.* London: Mosby.

Girkin, C. (2004). Primary open-angle glaucoma in African–Americans. *International Ophthalmic Clinics*, **44**(2), 43–60.

Glasgow, M. (2009). Glaucoma valvular devices.
Available at: http://www.medrounds.org/ocular-pathology-manual/2006/07/glaucoma-valvular-devices.html (last accessed August 2009).

Hoyng, P. and Kitazana, Y. (2002). Medical treatment of normal tension glaucoma. *Survey of Ophthalmology*, **47**(Suppl.1), S116–24.

Kanski, J. (2007). *Clinical Ophthalmology.* Oxford: Butterworth Heinemann.

Kwon, Y., Fingert, J. and Greenlee, E. (2007). A patient's guide to glaucoma.
Available at: http://www.medrounds.org/glaucoma-guide/2006/ (last accessed August 2009).

Loyo Berios, N. and, Blustein, J. (2007). Primary open-angle glaucoma and myopia: a narrative review. *Wisconsin Medical Journal*, **106**(2), 85–95.

Mercieca, K., Odogu, V., Fiebai, B., Arowolo, O. and Chukwuka, F. (2007). Comparison of central corneal thickness in a sub-Saharan cohort to African–Americans and Afro–Caribbeans. *Cornea*, **26**(5), 557–60.

National Institute for Health and Clinical Excellence (2007). Glaucoma draft scope for consultation. March 2007.
Available at: www.nice.org.uk/nicemedia/pdf/GlaucomaDraftScope.pdf (last accessed August 2009).

Noecker, R., Awadallah, N. and Kahook, M. (2007). Travoprost 0.004% / timolol 0.5% fixed combination. *Drugs of Today*, **43**(2), 77–83.

Pasquale, L., Kang, J., Manson, J., Willett, W., Rosner, B. and Hankinson, S. (2006). Prospective study of type 2 diabetes mellitus and the risk of primary open-angle glaucoma in women. *Ophthalmology*, **113**(7), 1081–86.

Quigley, H. and Broman, A. (2006). The number of people with glaucoma worldwide in 2010 and 2020. *British Journal of Ophthalmology*, **90**, 262–67.

Racette, L., Wilson, M., Zangwill, L., Weinreb, R. and Sample, P. (2003). Primary open-angle glaucoma in blacks: a review. *Survey of Ophthalmology*, **48**(3), 295–313.

Royal College of Ophthalmologists (2004). Statement on glaucoma. Richard Smith, Chairman Professional Standards Committee. Available at: http://www.rcophth.ac.uk/standards/statement-glaucoma.

Salmon, J.F. and Kanski, J.J. (2004). *Glaucoma: A Colour Manual of Diagnosis and Treatment.* Edinburgh: Butterworth Heinemann.

Sellers, D. (2008). Glaucoma, juvenile. Available at: http://emedicine.medscape.com/article/1207051-overview (last accessed August 2009).

Snell, R. and Lemp, M. (1998). *Clinical Anatomy of the Eye.* Oxford: Blackwell Science.

Sung, V., Koppens, J., Vernon, S., *et al.* (2006). Longitudinal glaucoma screening for siblings of patients with primary open-angle glaucoma: The Nottingham family glaucoma screening study. *British Journal of Ophthalmology*, **90**(1), 59–63.

Useful web resources

AOL video site

http://video.aol.com/

Search for trabeculectomy and the Ahmed valve. This site has a huge range of video clips.

eMedicine

http://emedicine.medscape.com/

Free Educational Publications International

http://www.eyepodvideo.org

Provides some 30 ophthalmic surgical videos for viewing.

Good Hope Hospital

http://www.goodhope.org.uk/

Good for glaucoma progression model, glaucoma progression text and trabeculectomy animation.

MedRounds

http://www.medrounds.org/

You will find Kwon et al.'s patient's guide to glaucoma and Glasgow's article on glaucoma valvular devices. There is further information on primary open-angle glaucoma, and the 'video pods' explore various aspects of surgery.

National Institute for Health and Clinical Excellence

http://www.nice.org.uk/

PubMed, Central National Institute of Health

http://www.pubmedcentral.nih.gov/

SELF TEST Answers on page 205

1. What percentage of people aged between 40 and 70 have primary open-angle glaucoma?

_____

2. What is the normal intraocular pressure?

_____

3. Name the two routes by which the aqueous is drained from the eye.

_____

4. What three tests should the community optometrist carry out to test for POAG?

_____

_____

5. Does ethnicity have any bearing on a person's chances of developing POAG?

_____

6. Why might the incidence of POAG be underestimated in black people?

_____

_____

7. What factor may distort intraocular pressure readings?

_____

8. Name a non-surgical intervention for POAG.

_____

9. How is normal tension glaucoma treated?

_____

_____

10. What are the symptoms of POAG?

_____

_____

_____

Chapter 9

Primary angle-closure glaucoma

Lynn Ring

Introduction

Primary acute angle-closure glaucoma (PAAC or PACG) is described by Kanski (2007) as 'occurring in anatomically disposed eyes without any other pathology'. This type of glaucoma occurs in hypermetropic (long-sighted) people, with shallow anterior chambers to their eyes. PAAC is caused solely by pupil block. Other causes of acute glaucoma symptoms include problems that are secondary to another eye condition, for example a sudden rise in eye pressure as a result of debris blocking the drainage angle following surgery or trauma. Qualified staff should be able to recognise the symptoms of this condition, and ensure that these patients receive prompt medical care.

Causes of the problem

Pupil block

The lens is the only structure in the body that continues to grow, and so in the older person it may be up to one-third larger than it was in youth. Hypermetropic (long-sighted) people may have a slightly more anteriorly placed lens, and have a shallow anterior chamber. The growing lens slowly begins to take up more space at the front of the eye, and moves forward a little and the drainage angle becomes progressively narrower. Eyes predisposed to this problem may have a smaller corneal diameter and axial length. Add to this the fact that in the older person there may be a tendency for the dilator muscle of the iris to atrophy slightly, causing the peripheral iris to bow forward. The lack of space at the front of the eye becomes critical. Posterior synaechiae may develop where the iris is in prolonged contact with the lens, and the development of areas of relative pupil block will cause the peripheral iris to balloon forward slightly and further obstruct the flow of aqueous from the posterior chamber as the peripheral iris now blocks the drainage angle.

Ageing

The condition affects women more than men for two reasons: firstly, most women have slightly shallower anterior chambers than men due to their generally slightly smaller eyes; secondly, women have a statistically longer life span in which to develop this disorder which is associated with maturity. Other risk factors include age, ethnicity and family history. The overall age for presentation is approximately 60 years. Asymptomatic patients are sometimes referred to the outpatient department by optometrists who have discovered one or more of the anatomical factors above, which might in time precipitate an attack of acute-angle closure. Primary acute angle-closure glaucoma is an acute emergency featuring sudden pain and visual loss.

Ethnicity

There is an increased risk of primary acute angle-closure glaucoma in South-East Asian and Chinese people (Congdon *et al.*, 1992) and Eskimos (Cox, 1984). In white people, it accounts for approximately 6% of all glaucoma cases (Salmon and Kanski, 2004).

Medicines

Certain drugs affect the pupil, for example, tricyclic antidepressants, antihistamines and phenothiazine antipsychotics. They can induce acute angle-closure in people who are predisposed to the condition (Salma, 2007).

Prodromal primary acute angle-closure

 Prior to developing an acute attack, a patient may have experienced episodes of headache, brow pain, haloes around lights, poor visual acuity and generally feeling unwell.

This happens particularly at night when poor lighting results in pupil dilation and consequent reduction in the entrance to the drainage angle. However these attacks tend to clear by the morning as the pupil mioses spontaneously during stage 3 sleep (sleep miosis/circadian miosis) (Noback *et al.* 2005) and the intraocular pressure returns to normal. If you suspect this has been happening to a friend or neighbour, you should refer the person urgently to the community optometrist for an ophthalmic opinion. At some future stage the person will develop a raised intraocular pressure that does not clear spontaneously. This may be brought on for the following reasons:

- **Going out in the dark** (e.g. visiting the cinema). Liew *et al.* (2008) state that 'pupil block, the underlying mechanism in acute-angle closure is believed to occur when the pupil is in a mid-dilated position, rather than a fully dilated position'.
- **Overwork, anxiety and stress** (and even heavy meals and general 'dissipation'!). These were suggested by Lyle *et al.* (1968) as contributory factors, but their ideas remain untested in the research literature, which cannot initiate a study to demonstrate whether these factors produce pupil dilatation.
- **Alcohol,** insofar as the effects of drinking large volumes of fluid are known to temporarily raise intraocular pressure (Susanna *et al.*, 2005).

Plateau iris

Plateau iris may cause primary acute-angle-closure glaucoma in younger people. The changes that begin to occur in the middle years of the gradual enlargement of the lens will precipitate an earlier angle closure in these more vulnerable eyes. Physiologically this person has either a slightly larger than average ciliary body or the ciliary body is situated in a slightly more anterior position. This has the effect of positioning the iris slightly more forward in relation to the drainage angle, resulting in an anterior chamber of normal depth, but with a very shallow drainage angle when assessed using the 'shadow' technique (Pearson, 2003). Kanski (2007) lists the treatment for this condition as laser iridotomy and pilocarpine 1%. The pilocarpine is necessary to miose the pupil and prevent 'plateau iris syndrome' when the pupil dilates and closes the iridotomy. Bruce *et al.* (2008) have published a well-illustrated article on plateau iris.

To do ...

Find out why a patient who had prodromal glaucoma symptoms might complain of haloes and blurred vision.

Symptoms of primary acute angle-closure

 Pain: This is sudden and extreme with an onset of between 30 and 60 minutes, and is felt particularly around the brow on the affected side.

 Rapid drop in visual acuity: This is seriously reduced, often to as low as 6/60 or even 'count fingers'.

 Haloes around lights: These may be mentioned as a symptom of the oedematous cornea.

 General unwellness: The patient feels generally very unwell, often experiencing nausea, possibly vomiting. Vomiting and prostration may be so severe as to cause confusion with gastroenteritis. Skuta (1994) suggests that the abrupt rise in intraocular pressure may produce autonomic stimulation and associated nausea, vomiting, bradycardia and diaphoresis (sweating).

The following signs may be observed by the health professional:

 Crimson red conjunctiva, sometimes showing chemosis, with a crimson flush around the cornea.

 Hazy cornea due to oedema.

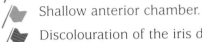 Shallow anterior chamber.

 Discolouration of the iris due to ischaemia caused by the raised pressure.

 Fixed, semi-dilated pupil, looking slightly oval in shape.

Engorged iris vessels.

Intraocular pressure is extremely high – often as high as 70 mmHg. Be very careful when measuring this, as the cornea is very oedematous, and will abrade easily.

The triage nurse in any minor injuries or accident or eye department must inform the medical staff immediately of any patient with suspected acute glaucoma so that treatment can commence as soon as possible. There may only be a short period from the onset of this condition to treat, otherwise the patient may suffer irreversible visual loss in the affected eye.

Treatment priorities

These are to:

- record any allergies and other medications.
- reduce intraocular pressure
- relieve symptoms such as nausea and vomiting
- reduce anxiety
- suppress inflammation
- prepare for self-care at home following treatment.

Nursing care

Intravenous and topical medications are prepared ready for and given on prescription. However the nurse can initiate certain actions:

- Lie the patient supine, allowing the lens to shift backwards, in a darkened, quiet room if possible.
- Provide a vomit bowl and tissues. Mouthwash may be appreciated if the patient is vomiting.
- Support the patient by a reassuring presence.
- Cold compresses may help the pain.
- While the patient is resting, ensure further equipment and medications are on hand if required.
- Prepare the intravenous acetazolamide 500 mg with the equipment for intravenous cannulation.

- Cannulate the patient (if you are competent to do this).
- Prepare an intravenous antiemetic if required.

Topical medications may also be prescribed by the ophthalmologist, including:

- dexamethasone (Maxidex™) anti-inflammatory drops
- ocular hypotensive beta-blockers such as timolol (Timoptol™)
- apraclonidine (Iopidine™), a selective sympathomimetic
- pilocarpine 2% (miotic) to the fellow eye (possibly; see below).

N.B. Due to iris ischaemia there is no place for 'intensive' miotic therapy to the affected eye. If the intraocular pressure exceeds 30 mmHg then the sphincter muscle is usually ischaemic and unable to respond to miotics (Salmon and Kanski, 2004).

Explain to the patient every intervention and treatment as this condition is very worrying, debilitating and exhausting. The patient, who feels very ill, might otherwise take exception to the treatments and become uncooperative if the interventions are not understood.

Ocular examination by the ophthalmologist will include further checking of the intraocular pressure, gonioscopy and optic disc assessment. However the ophthalmologist will not be able to examine and assess the drainage angle until the cornea has cleared sufficiently. Make sure that the gonioscopy lens, local anaesthetic and methyl cellulose eye-drops are readily available.

To do ...

Check for information about acetazolamide (Diamox™).

Note the side effects of this medication.

What advice should you give your patient regarding side effects?

 Never forget that 1g of acetazolamide is the total recommended dose in 24 hours.

Very occasionally this is exceeded (on consultant instruction only, after you have informed him or her that the patient has already received the maximum dose).

After 1 hour re-check the intraocular pressure. If it has reduced to below 30 mmHg, the ophthalmologist may prescribe pilocarpine 2% to reduce the pupil size and draw the drainage angle open.

 If the intraocular pressure has not reduced below 35 mmHg, inform the ophthalmologist.

Persistent raised pressure may require the use of mannitol 20% to create a forced diuresis and lower the intraocular pressure. This is calculated at 1–1.5 g per kilogram of body weight given as prescribed via an intravenous giving set.

Oral glycerol 50% solution is very rarely used these days, but may be ordered at 1 g per kg body weight diluted with fresh lemon or lime juice.

The patient is likely to take home oral and topical medications to control the intraocular pressure while the acute episode is settling and the cornea is clearing. They will need a Nd:YAG laser iridotomy once the cornea is clear and the iris congestion is reduced. This may not be possible until 24–48 hours after the initial attack but does depend on the severity of this episode. Give the patient and relative (if available) accurate information and guidance about caring for their eye at home.

Follow-up

A follow-up appointment will be arranged within 48 hours to facilitate laser treatment, but it is likely that the patient will return the following day for further examination and treatment if possible. However it is appropriate to carry out a prophylactic iridotomy on the fellow eye if the patient is able to cooperate. Remember it is unusual to have different anatomy in each eye and therefore the fellow eye is at risk of developing an acute-angle closure. Prophylactic pilocarpine 2% drops used to be provided for the unaffected eye pending laser treatment, but their use has become controversial. Obviously pilocarpine mioses the pupil and pulls the peripheral iris away from the drainage angle. However, Mohammed *et al.* (2001) point out that there have been a number of case reports regarding an additional, paradoxical effect of pilocarpine – it causes shallowing of the anterior chamber and potentially causes angle closure in compromised eyes.

Peripheral iridotomy

Peripheral iridotomy is advocated as the initial treatment for acute-angle-closure glaucoma (Salmon and Kanski, 2004) but they identify that this may be difficult in the acute phase due to corneal oedema and iris congestion. The purpose of the laser iridotomy is to re-establish the link between the posterior chamber and the anterior chamber by making a 'hole' in the iris fibres. The patient needs to have a full explanation and full information in order to give informed consent. The site for the peripheral iridotomy is usually between the 11 o'clock and 2 o'clock positions. This sits under the upper lid and can be seen as red reflex when patent. If the iridotomy is unsuccessful (in 25% of cases according to Kanski, 2007) then the patient may require long-term treatment (e.g. with latanoprost) or proceed to trabeculectomy.

Primary acute angle-closure glaucoma

Primary acute angle-closure glaucoma only exists when the primary angle-closure has resulted in optic nerve damage and visual field loss (Kanski, 2007). It is interesting to note that worldwide cases of acute closed-angle glaucoma have declined following the increased availability of cataract surgery. Fraser and Wormald (2008) used UK Hospital Episode Statistics to explore this trend within UK society, and noted that a 52% increase in cataract surgery has been accompanied by a reduction in the number of trabeculectomies by 50%. Laser trabeculectomies are down by 60% and laser peripheral iridectomies by 30%. However, they caution that these figures may not be entirely accurate because, for example, the advent of prostaglandin eye-drops has not been taken into consideration.

To do ...

Ask your senior nurses or medical colleagues about treatment for primary acute angle-closure glaucoma. Find out the protocols within your unit.

Visual prognosis

Aung *et al.* (2001) studied a Singaporean population and found that 38% of patients following primary acute angle-closure had visual field defects post treatment and could therefore be deemed to have developed primary acute angle-closure glaucoma. But they caution that some of this damage may have existed prior to their acute episode.

There is clearly a role for preventive ophthalmology in the detection and treatment of eyes at risk with shallow anterior chambers and narrow angles before they develop primary-angle closure. This again endorses the health professional's role in promoting the value of regular visits to a local optometrist to our client group.

Long-term prognosis

Other pathological conditions may arise as a result of an acute attack. There can be iris atrophy including posterior synaechiae between the pupil margin and the anterior lens capsule, cataract formation including white flakes on the lens surface (glaukomflecken), peripheral synaechiae, and optic disc cupping. These are all as a result of very high intraocular pressure and disturbance of aqueous circulation.

Routine pupil dilatation in the eye clinic

Question: Can you think of a **potential** risk factor that occurs every day in an eye unit with patients who have shallow anterior chambers, narrow angles or who are hypermetropes?

Answer: Nurses will dilate patients who come to the eye clinic, theoretically unintentionally performing a provocation test. This is when the patient has their pupils dilated and intraocular pressure checked to ascertain whether the intraocular pressure is elevated when dilated.

Question: Should you always check for a shallow anterior chamber and whether a patient is hypermetropic before administering dilating eye-drops?

Answer: Not necessarily. Pandit and Taylor (2000) found that the risk of inducing acute glaucoma with mydriasis using tropicamide (Mydriacyl) alone is close to zero (no case having been identified).

Patel *et al.* (1995) in a study to examine the incidence of primary acute angle-closure glaucoma after pharmacological dilatation reported that of 5,307 residents examined in the Baltimore eye study, not one developed acute glaucoma, although 38 of them were judged to have occludable angles on the basis of gonioscopy examination. Liew *et al.* (2006) evaluated worldwide studies and found the risk of developing primary acute angle-closure glaucoma as ranging from 1 in 20,000 of the population to 1 in 2400 in Malay Singaporean people, who are particularly susceptible. Liew *et al.* (2006) concluded that 'pupil dilatation is important for thorough fundoscopy, and the risk of precipitating primary acute angle-closure glaucoma with the routine use of mydriatics is close to zero'.

For personal interest and future development

If you do decide to develop skills in the assessment of anterior chamber depth, this should be an agreed part of a personal development plan, and ideally your skills should be built and formally evaluated as part of your work in a glaucoma clinic.

You might like to read the illustrated material found on Dr H.D. Riley's Clinical Science site, on how to estimate anterior chamber depth using an ophthalmoscope. A more in-depth explanation is given by Pearson (2003).

However, as you will discover while reading the next chapter, glaucoma is an extremely complex area of study and practice. Information has been presented to help you develop clinical proficiency, but if you intend to specialise in this area, and develop clinical expertise, it would be appropriate to study this subject at master's level.

References and further reading

Aung, T., Looi, A. and Chew, P. (2001). The visual field following acute primary angle closure glaucoma. *Acta Ophthalmologica Scandinavica*, **79**,(3), 298–300.

Bruce, A., Day, J., McKay, D. and Swann, P. (2008). Plateau iris syndrome. *Optician*, February 2008. Available at: http://www.opticianonline.net/Articles/2008/02/15/20385/Plateau + iris.htm (last accessed August 2009).

Congdon, N., Wang, F. and Tielsch, J. (1992). Issues in the epidemiology and population-based screening of primary angle-closure glaucoma. *Surveys in Ophthalmology*, **36**, 411–23.

Cox, J. (1984). Angle closure glaucoma amongst the Alaskan Eskimos. *Glaucoma*, 6, 335–37.

Darkeh, A. and Silverberg, M. (2006). Glaucoma. Acute angle closure. Available at: http://emedicine.medscape.com/article/798811-overview (last accessed August 2009).

Fraser, S. and Wormald, R. (2008). Hospital episode statistics and changing trends in glaucoma surgery. *Eye*, 22(1), 3–7.

Kanski, J. (2007). *Clinical Ophthalmology*. Oxford: Butterworth Heinemann.

Liew, G., Mitchell, P. and Wang, J. (2006). Fundoscopy: to dilate or not to dilate? (Editorial). *British Medical Journal*, **332**, 3.

Lyle, T., Cross, A. and Cook, C. (1968). *May and Worth's Diseases of the Eye*. London: Balliere Tindall and Cassell.

Mohammed, Q., Fahey, D. and Manners, R. (2001). Angle closure in the fellow eye with prophylactic pilocarpine treatment. *British Journal of Ophthalmology*, **85**, 1260.

Noback R., Strominger N., Demarest R., Raggiero D., 2005. *The human nervous system: Structure and function*. New Jersey, USA:.Humana Press,

Pandit, R. and Taylor, R. (2000). Mydriasis and glaucoma: exploding the myth. A systemic review. *Diabetic Medicine: A Journal of the British Diabetic Association*, **17**(10), 693–99.

Patel, K., Jaritt, J., Tielsch, J., *et al.* (1995). Incidence of acute angle-closure glaucoma after pharmacological mydriasis. *American Journal of Ophthalmology*, **120**(6), 709–19.

Pearson, R. (2003). Optometric grading scales. *Optometry Today*, October 17, 39–42. Available at: http://www.optometry.co.uk/articles.php?keyword = optometric + grading + scales&author = Pearson&year = 2003&Submit2 = Submit (last accessed June 2009).

Salma, R. (2007). Antispasmodics: choice, mode of action and prescribing issues. *Nurse Prescriber*, 5(11), 500–05.

Salmon, J. and Kanski, J. (2004). *Glaucoma: A Colour Manual of Diagnosis and Treatment*. Edinburgh: Butterworth Heinemann.

Skuta, G. (1994). The angle closure glaucomas. In: S. Podos and M. Yanoff (eds) *Textbook of Ophthalmology*. London: Mosby.

Susanna, R., Vessani, R., Sakata, L., Zacarias, L. and Hatanaka, M. (2005). The relationship between intraocular pressure peak in the water drinking test and visual field progression in glaucoma. *British Journal of Ophthalmology*, 89(10),1298–3001.

Useful web resources

Dr H.D. Riley's Clinical Science II & III (Indiana University School of Optometry)
http://www.opt.indiana.edu/riley/rileyshome.html
For information on direct ophthalmoscopy.

Good Hope Hospital
http://www.goodhope.org.uk
For more on angle closure glaucoma.

Optician Online
http://www.opticianonline.net/Home/Default.aspx
For more on plateau iris syndrome.

Optometry Today
http://www.optometry.co.uk/articles.php
Look for Pearson's article on optometric grading scales.

SELF TEST Answers on page 205

1. Which group of people have eyes that are anatomically disposed to develop primary angle-closure?

2. Name two factors that contribute to pupil block in primary angle-closure.

3. What is a prodromal attack of primary angle-closure?

4. Name two symptoms of primary angle-closure.

5. If you examined the eye of a patient with primary angle-closure with a pen torch, what diagnostic signs might you detect?

6. What drug is normally given intravenously?

7. What is the laser treatment for this condition called?

8. Is it dangerous to dilate a patient's eye with tropicamide (Mydriacyl™) without checking the anterior chamber depth first?

Chapter 10

The secondary glaucomas

Lynn Ring

This third chapter on glaucoma contains brief information on some of the rarer, more complex glaucomas. It expected that you will use it:

- as a reference resource when you come across one of these secondary glaucomas
- to build up your knowledge if you are regularly involved in glaucoma clinics
- as introductory information if you are seeking to expand your role within the eye department's glaucoma services
- in the ophthalmic theatre, to explain some of the procedures you will be involved with, or a patient's relevant ophthalmic history.

All secondary glaucomas develop as a result of another eye condition. Many eye disorders, injuries, operations of the eye and even medical treatments can lead to increased intraocular pressure and potential optic nerve damage. Diagnosis and treatment of the root cause may be sufficient to return the intraocular pressure to normal and prevent lasting damage. For ease of understanding, they have been divided into various groups.

Secondary glaucomas and the lens

Phacolytic glaucoma

If a cataract is not operated on when the vision becomes hazy and is left to develop, it may become hyper-mature and begin to liquefy. Eventually lens proteins leak out into the anterior chamber of the eye, causing obstruction within the trabecular meshwork and anterior uveitis. This is very occasionally seen in UK hospitals, among patients who have hitherto been terrified of surgery. Treatment is with steroid eye-drops to reduce the inflammation, as well as patient support and counselling, followed by cataract extraction.

Phacomorphic glaucoma

A swollen (intumescent) cataract takes up sufficient space to block aqueous from circulating through the pupil into the drainage angle (pupil block). This has a secondary consequence whereby the trapped aqueous causes the base of the iris to balloon forward, resulting in an acute-angle closure. Sometimes this occurs in elderly long-sighted people with a relatively small eye. As a cataract develops, the lens swells naturally and takes up more space in an already shallow anterior chamber. Fewer elderly people are affected nowadays as a result of free eye tests in the UK and generally faster provision of cataract surgery by the NHS. Phacomorphic glaucoma is also a particular complication of traumatic injury to the lens capsule, in which aqueous is able to enter and causes swelling of the lens. Treatment is with ocular hypotensive drops such as acetazolamide (Diamox™), mannitol and urgent cataract extraction.

Lens dislocation glaucoma

A lens dislocated into the anterior segment of the eye may cause an acute pupil block, leading to a secondary angle closure with a sudden rise in intraocular pressure. It can be the result of weak lens zonules giving way, for example in a person with Marfan syndrome. It can also occur following blunt eye trauma. Treatment involves initial medical control of the intraocular pressure followed by surgical removal of the lens. Kanski (2007) suggests that if the fellow eye might have a similar attack, a prophylactic laser iridotomy is indicated.

Note:

The lens does not always dislocate into the anterior chamber. Subluxation is an incomplete dislocation as some lens zonules remain intact.

To do ...

Ask senior nurses in your accident and emergency department whether they remember a patient with lens-induced acute glaucoma. What happened and why did it happen?

Eye injuries and glaucoma

Red cell glaucoma

This may occur following a blunt-force trauma to the eye, causing a hyphaema in the anterior chamber. Obviously the hyphaema will vary in size according to the severity of the injury, but Kanski (2007) states that if the bleeding fills half or less of the anterior chamber, then there is a 4% risk of raised intraocular pressure. If the blood fills more than half of the anterior chamber, there is an 85% risk of raised intraocular pressure. The initial rise in intraocular pressure is associated with blood cells temporarily blocking the trabecular meshwork. Following a large hyphaema, however, damage may be caused to the trabecular meshwork in the long term, as the trabecular endothelial cells phagocytose the red cell residues; the accumulation of iron from the haem cells is toxic, so the endothelial cells may eventually degenerate and fibrose, contributing to an outflow obstruction (Sehu and Lee, 2005). A large blood clot in the anterior chamber can trigger a pupil-block glaucoma and other major ocular complications.

 Secondary bleeds may occur, usually more severely than the original bleed in the 3–5 days following the original injury, possibly as a result of the body's normal thrombolysis of the original clotted haemorrhage. If the intraocular pressure rises as a result of either the original or any secondary bleed, and is not adequately monitored and controlled, then the optic nerve may suffer some permanent damage.

Initial treatment is aimed at preventing secondary haemorrhage. Walton *et al.* (2002) state that topical steroids will reduce ocular inflammation and reduce the risk of secondary haemorrhage. The pupil is kept dilated, to 'splint' it in position, thus reducing the risk of secondary bleeding from the iris or ciliary body.

Ghost cell glaucoma

This type of glaucoma is characterised by the presence of old red blood cells that have degenerated into khaki-coloured cells in the aqueous or vitreous and which may settle in the drainage angle. It may be of traumatic or non-traumatic origin (Zimmerman and Kooner, 2001). To be a little more specific, it may follow, for example, a spontaneous vitreous haemorrhage, trauma to the eye, or vitreoretinal surgery. Treatment is medical, but if the condition fails to respond then surgery may be necessary.

Angle recession glaucoma

Blunt-force trauma may trigger angle recession, a complex injury to the ciliary body. It has been described in detail by Sullivan (2006) who suggests that angle recession is a common finding after contusion trauma, and that in patients with identified angle trauma, lengthy follow-up is justified due to the risk of delayed, asymptomatic glaucoma developing. Medical therapy with eye-drops is the initial treatment, but the patient's response may be variable, so laser and surgical options may need to be considered in the long run.

Glaucoma associated with retinal ischaemia

Neovascular glaucoma

Neovascular glaucoma is the current term for a collection of problems that were historically referred to as *haemorrhagic* glaucoma, *thrombotic* glaucoma, *congestive* glaucoma, *rubeotic* glaucoma and *diabetic haemorrhagic* glaucoma. Kanski (2007) states that causes of ischaemic retina and consequently neovascularisation glaucoma are: central retinal vein occlusion (36%), proliferative diabetic retinopathy (32%) and various other conditions such as central retinal artery occlusion, longstanding retinal detachment and chronic intraocular inflammation.

Neovascular glaucoma is a relatively common eye problem with a range of causes, all having at their root severe, chronic retinal ischaemia. The hypoxic retina produces growth factors to try to re-vascularise the hypoxic retinal tissue. The most significant of these is currently thought to be vascular endothelial growth factor (VEGF). Where the circulation to the retina is particularly poor, VEGF will tend to be concentrated in the blood vessels of the posterior iris, new growth from which will initially appear at the pupil margin, and gradually vascularise the anterior iris and eventually the drainage angle. Ultimately this will block the aqueous outflow (rubeosis iridis).

In the early stages of neovascular glaucoma the drainage angle is open, but if the condition is left to progress, a secondary angle closure will result. *Rubeosis iridis* can be prevented by pan-retinal laser photocoagulation of the ischaemic retina, with the intention of causing new-vessel regression. When successful, this treatment prevents many of the problems associated with an ischaemic retina, of which rubeosis iridis is just one. Clearly, careful medical management of any underlying systemic disease related to the ischaemic problem within the eye is essential; as Blanc *et al.* (2004) point out, people with neovascular glaucoma historically demonstrate a markedly reduced life expectancy.

Treatment options for neovascular glaucoma include:

- Pan-retinal laser photocoagulation: As mentioned above, initially the drainage angle is open, so progression may be averted by pan-retinal laser photocoagulation. However, if the disease is left to progress, the drainage angle will become progressively more closed.

- Eye-drops: Clearly in the early stages, when patients have iris and angle neovascularisation but no peripheral anterior synaechiae at the drainage angle, the glaucoma may be controlled with topical ocular hypotensive eye-drops that reduce the intraocular pressure.

- Trabeculectomy (or implantation of a device such as the Ahmed™ valve): This will provide an alternative route for aqueous drainage and may be helpful if the condition has progressed.

- Photodynamic therapy: This has been used successfully for a number of years to obliterate anterior segment neovascularisation (Parodi *et al.*, 2008).

- Trans-scleral diode laser photocoagulation: This is used in people who do not respond to other treatments and whose vision is already seriously reduced. The aim is to destroy part of the ciliary body to reduce aqueous production. Repeated treatments may be needed. What little visual acuity remains is likely to be preserved, but it can result in hypotony (a very soft eye) and phthiasis (a shrunken, unsightly blind eye). Asari and Gandhewar (2007) studied the long-term efficacy and visual acuity following this procedure. They concluded that it was highly effective and safe for various types of glaucoma and its use could be extended to eyes with good vision.

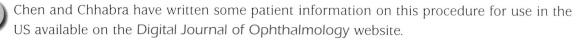

  Chen and Chhabra have written some patient information on this procedure for use in the US available on the *Digital Journal of Ophthalmology* website.

- Cyclocryothermy: This is the application of extreme cold. Temperatures as low as −80°C are applied to the eye tissue lying above the ciliary body. This destroys the capacity of the ciliary body to produce normal quantities of aqueous fluid. It is not generally attempted until the patient's vision is extremely poor and other methods of controlling the glaucoma have proved inadequate or the patient has a painful blind eye. It is performed with the patient lying on his or her back and requires local anaesthesia. An initial eye-drop of local anaestheticis used, often followed by a retrobulbar or peribulbar injection. Following the cryothermy procedure, a subconjunctival steroid injection is usually given to reduce inflammation. Atropine is often given to reduce pain from ciliary muscle spasm. The patient must be monitored for excessive pain due to possible increased intraocular pressure, and normally continues with antihypertensive eye-drops.

End-stage neovascular glaucoma (absolute glaucoma)

This form of glaucoma is beyond any further treatment. A topical steroid is used to reduce inflammation and inhibit cell proliferation. Topical atropine 1% is given to decrease ocular congestion and pain. If this fails to provide the appropriate pain relief then patients may choose to proceed to enucleation, as the pain from this condition is intractable (Khan *et al.*, 2006).

> ## To do ...
>
> Find out what '100-day' glaucoma means from your senior colleagues. How is this normally prevented?

Steroid-induced glaucoma

The use of topical steroids is common in ophthalmic practice. However, these should *always* be used cautiously.

Although the mechanism is not fully understood, the use of topical steroids for inflammatory conditions, either as treatment in acute episodes or for prophylactic prevention in the postoperative period, can provoke a high intraocular pressure in 'steroid responders'. For this reason steroid drops should be used with caution in people known to have primary open-angle glaucoma (and their immediate relatives). All patients on steroid eye-drops should be warned about relevant symptoms, which include acute onset of pain, increased redness and reduced vision, and they should be instructed about what to do should these arise.

Note:

It is common practice to use steroids after cataract surgery in people with open-angle glaucoma to reduce intraocular inflammation for the short postoperative period – some surgeons use diclofenac as an alternative. It is important to check and record the intraocular pressure before commencing steroid eye treatments.

Inflammatory glaucoma

This secondary group of glaucomas is associated with intraocular inflammation that arises idiopathically, or as a result of trauma or systemic disease. The intraocular pressure may rise due to inflammation, causing acute trabeculitis or blockage of the drainage angle with inflammatory debris.

Anterior uveitis

Posterior synaechiae that form as a result of inflammation may cause 'pupil block'. Without adequate treatment, peripheral anterior synaechiae may develop following repeated episodes of acute anterior uveitis. This is the reason for intensive pupil dilatation and nursing and medical efforts to ensure that patients with anterior uveitis are always adequately dilated before they leave the eye department. Kanski (2007) stipulates that short-acting mydriatics allow the pupil some movement and thus avoid posterior synaechiae in the dilated position.

In posterior synaechiae pupil block, medical treatment and laser iridotomy is required and some patients may require further surgical intervention if angle closure is permanent. An inflamed iris is easily stuck to the trabecular meshwork and iridocorneal contact becomes permanent.

Note:

Raised intraocular pressure is not a diagnostic feature of anterior uveitis, for example, because initially the patient may have normal or subnormal intraocular pressure due to ciliary body shut-down. It is more likely that a secondary glaucoma will occur later due to obstruction of aqueous outflow when the initial inflammation is settling and ciliary function returning to normal. However, intraocular pressure is measured routinely at all the patient's attendances to monitor for potential changes.

To do ...

What is iris bombee? Discuss it with your colleagues.

Syndromes associated with inflammatory glaucoma

Fuchs' uveitis syndrome

Fuchs' uveitis is an insidious onset, unilateral, chronic anterior segment inflammation. Heterochromia is considered an important feature of this condition, but it is not present in all patients. The most common complication is cataract formation, but secondary open-angle and closed-angle glaucoma can occur. Bonfioli *et al.* (2005) identified that the iris and trabecular meshwork may show abnormal vessels and synaechiae. Gupta (2004) theorised that trabecular inflammation might produce sclerosis, leading to closed-angle glaucoma. Patients with Fuchs' uveitis are at a 10–15% greater risk of developing open-angle glaucoma (Riordan Eva *et al.*, 2003) and these patients are monitored regularly.

Posner–Schlossman syndrome

Green (2007) describes a patient who was initially misdiagnosed with acute glaucoma, and defines Posner–Schlossman syndrome as 'a recurrent ocular inflammatory disease, diagnosis of which can be challenging'. The raised intraocular pressure is accompanied by or followed within a few days by a mild, often symptomless uveal inflammation. Treatment is medical, to reduce the inflammation and intraocular pressure. Patients present with mild unilateral pain, photophobia and blurred vision. Jager and Lamkin (2005) stated that these patients are often 20–50 years old. Around 33% of them have heterochromia, and their pupils may be unequally dilated, with the affected eye having reduced accommodation. They believe the problem to be associated with infection by varicella zoster virus.

Attacks are experienced in both eyes at different times. Treatment is to reduce inflammation and intraocular pressure medically. Attacks occur at lengthening intervals, but follow-up monitoring of intraocular pressure, optic discs and visual fields is essential as all these patients are more liable to develop primary open-angle glaucoma (POAG). Jap *et al.* (2001) demonstrated that the risk more than doubles 10 years after developing the syndrome.

Miscellaneous secondary open-angle glaucomas

Pigment dispersion syndrome

Pigment dispersion syndrome (or PDS) is a bilateral condition, the result of the posterior iris rubbing against the lens zonules, causing the release of pigment granules. The aqueous circulation disperses these granules throughout the anterior chamber. They settle on the various structures, particularly the trabecular meshwork, where they lie both on the surface and inside and cause obstruction, damage and scarring (Kanski, 2007). This condition features typical vertical spindle-shaped deposits on the corneal endothelium, known as Krukenberg spindles. Armstrong (2009) gives a detailed explanation and an image of this diagnostic feature.

Siddiqui *et al.* (2003) state that the syndrome occurs more frequently in males than in females and up to 10% of patients who have it will progress to chronic open-angle glaucoma after 5 years (15% at 15 years). Therefore it is important to maintain regular follow-up for these patients in the eye clinic. Haynes *et al.* (1992) demonstrated that in some people with the syndrome, vigorous or strenuous physical activity precipitates release of pigment granules, resulting in increased intraocular pressure. They demonstrated that pilocarpine eye-drops could inhibit the problem by restricting iris movement. The treatment regimen is similar to that of POAG initially using medical therapies but more often than not it requires laser trabeculoplasty and trabeculectomy.

Pseudoexfoliation

Pseudoexfoliation syndrome of the eye is now believed to be an ocular manifestation of a systemic disorder of the basement membrane in epithelial cells (Schlotzer and Naumann, 2006). In the affected individual's eye, the ageing epithelial cells produce a grey-white material, which is deposited around the posterior and anterior chambers on the anterior surface of the lens capsule, the zonules, the iris and the trabecular meshwork. If the pupil is dilated, this material can be seen on slit lamp examination at the pupil margins and on the anterior lens surface. Transillumination shows pupil atrophy. Gonioscopy shows trabecular hyperpigmentation, particularly inferiorly, and has a patchy distribution unlike that of pigment dispersion syndrome.

Pseudoexfoliation is more common in females than in males, but males are more likely to develop chronic open-angle glaucoma, if affected. Again the risk of developing chronic glaucoma is 5% at 5 years but 15% at 10 years. Patients with pseudoexfoliation glaucoma in one eye and pseudoexfoliation in the fellow eye are at 50% risk of developing glaucoma in the second eye within 5 years (Salmon and Kanski, 2003).

Treatment options remain similar to those for POAG and medical therapy has initial success, but it is more likely that these patients will need further surgical interventions.

Conclusions

A new member of staff needs to understand the basic components and some of the more common conditions associated with raised intraocular pressure. They can build upon that knowledge base as experience develops. Glaucoma is a diverse and fascinating group of optic neuropathies that seems to be continually evolving in terms of treatment options and patient interactions.

Experienced nurses can develop their practice to include examination of patients using the slit lamp, measuring intraocular pressure with Goldmann applanation tonometry, optic disc assessment and visual field measurement and interpretation. Nurses will continue to develop, while remembering and building upon a nursing background and philosophy of caring for the individual. It is possible to develop the nursing role to include individual enhanced skills, such as intraocular pressure measurement, and to develop a phasing clinic or intraocular pressure clinic where patients newly commenced on treatment or with changed treatment regimens can come into a nursing clinic for the intraocular pressure measurement and general review.

Further to intraocular pressure clinics, nurses are working at advanced practice level and undertaking educational programmes to first degree and master's level to enable them to undertake full review of new patients in glaucoma clinics, including initiating treatment regimens or discharging patients back to the community appropriately. They also carry out follow-up clinics including interpretation of visual fields and optic disc assessment.

Nurses are undertaking independent non-medical prescribing modules to support their practice. They are developing new ways of working to support patients and enable their eye departments to deliver high standards of service to patients and to achieve government initiated modernisation. These nurses are working as autonomous practitioners within their local glaucoma services supported by appropriate advanced-level educational programmes and their colleagues to ensure that patients benefit from seeing the right person, at the right time and often in the right place.

To do ...

Do you have nurse-led intraocular pressure clinics? If so, ask the nurse what preparation they undertook to enhance their role. What personal development plans do you have for when you become an experienced ophthalmic nurse?

References and further reading

Armstrong, T. (2009). Krukenberg's spindle.
Available at: http://www.krukenbergs-spindle.co.uk/Krukenbergs_Spindle.htm (last accessed August 2009).

Asari, E. and Gandhewar, J. (2007). Long-term efficacy and visual acuity following trans-scleral diode laser photocoagulation in cases of refractory and non-refractory glaucoma. *Eye*, 21(7), 936–40.

Blanc, J., Molteno, A., Fuller, J., Bevin, T. and Herbison, P. (2004). Life expectancy of patients with glaucoma drained by Molteno implants. *Clinical and Experimental Ophthalmology,* 32(4), 360–63.

Bonfioli, A., Curis, A. and Orefice, F. (2005). Fuchs' heterochromic cyclitis. *Seminars in Ophthalmology*, 20(3), 143–46.

Green, R. (2007). Possner–Schlossman syndrome – glaucomatocyclitic crisis. *Clinical and Experimental Optometry: Journal of the Australian Optometric Association*, 90(1), 53–56.

Gupta, D. (2004). *Glaucoma Diagnosis and Management*. Philadelphia: Lippincott, Williams and Wilkins.

Haynes, W., Johnson, A. and Alward, W. (1992). Effects of jogging exercise on patients with pigment dispersal syndrome and pigmentary glaucoma. *Ophthalmology*, 99(7), 1096–1103.

Jager, R. and Lamkin, J. (2005). *The Massachusetts Eye and Ear Infirmary Review Manual for Ophthalmology,* 3rd edn. Philadelphia: Lippincott, Williams and Wilkins.

Jap, A., Sivakumar, M. and Chee, S. (2001). Is Possner-Schlossman syndrome benign? *Ophthalmology*, 180(5), 913–18.

Kanski, J. (2007). *Clinical Ophthalmology*. Oxford: Butterworth Heinemann.

Khan, I., Hasanee, K. and Khan, B. (2006). Glaucoma, neovascular.
Available at: http://emedicine.medscape.com/article/1205736-overview (last accessed August 2009).

Parodi, M., Iacono, P. and Ranalico, G. (2008). Verteporfin photodynamic therapy for anterior segment neovascularisation secondary to ischaemic central retinal vein occlusion. *Clinical and Experimental Ophthalmology*, 36(3), 232–37.

Riordan-Eva, P., Whitcher, J., Vaughan, D. and Asbury, T. (2003). *Vaughan and Asbury's General Ophthalmology*. Maidenhead: McGraw-Hill Professional.

Salmon, J. and Kanski, J. (2003). *Glaucoma: A Colour Manual of Diagnosis and Treatment*. Oxford: Butterworth Heineman.

Schlotzer-Schrehardt, U. and Naumann, G. (2006). Ocular and systemic pseudoexfoliation syndrome. *American Journal of Ophthalmology*, 141(5), 921–37.

Sehu, W. and Lee, W. (2005). *Ophthalmic Pathology: An Illustrated Guide for Clinicians*. Oxford: Blackwell BMJ Books.

Siddiqui, Y., Ten Hulzen, R., Cameron, D., Hodge, D. and Johnson, D. (2003). What is the risk of developing pigmentary glaucoma from pigment dispersal syndrome? *American Journal of Ophthalmology*, 135(6), 794–99.

Sullivan, B. (2006). Glaucoma, angle recession. emedicine from WebMD.
Available at: http://www.emedicine.com/oph/topic121.htm (last accessed August 2009).

Walton, W., Von Hagen, S., Grigorian, S. and Zarbin, M. (2002). Management of traumatic hyphaema. *Survey of Ophthalmology*, 47(4), 1372–78.

Zimmerman, T. and Kooner, T. (2001). *Clinical Pathways in Glaucoma*. New York: Thieme.

Useful web resources

Digital Journal of Ophthalmology
http://www.djo.harvard.edu/
Look for the article by Chen and Chhabra on diode laser trans-scleral cyclophotocoagulation.

emedicine from WebMD
http://www.webmd.com/
For more on neovascular and angle recession glaucoma see the articles by Khan and Sullivan, respectively.

Handbook of Ocular Disease Management
http://www.revoptom.com/HANDBOOK/hbhome.htm
Search for information on pigment dispersion syndrome.

Krukenberg's spindle
http://www.krukenbergs-spindle.co.uk/
The Encyclopaedia of Surgery
http://www.surgeryencyclopedia.com/
Further information on secondary glaucomas and a guide for patients and carers on cyclocryotherapy.

SELF TEST Answers on page 206

1. Name a secondary glaucoma that may arise as a result of a hyper-mature or intumescent cataract.

_____

2. Name two secondary glaucomas that can occur as a result of blunt trauma to the eye.

_____

_____

3. Name two subtypes of neovascular glaucoma.

_____

_____

4. What is the name of the group of patients in whom steroid-induced glaucoma can provoke raised intraocular pressure?

_____

5. Anterior uveitis can give rise to what kind of glaucoma?

_____

6. PDS is short for which secondary glaucoma?

_____

7. Is pseudexfoliation more common in men or women?

_____

Chapter 11

Retinal problems

Dorothy Field

This chapter will ask you a lot of questions, and take you a long time to complete, so only aim to tackle one section at a time. It is a good idea to write your answers down as you go to create your own reference resource. As with the other chapters, do check out your understanding with either your mentor or a nurse who specialises in this field, and start to take particular notice of the patients with retinal conditions that you encounter in clinical practice. This is a large and very complex area of practice, and only the main areas can be covered here.

Retinal detachment

Refer back to the diagrams and text concerned with the retina in Chapter 2. You will note that because of the way the embryo developed, the retina originally consists of two layers, the nervous layer and the pigment layer, that bond together as the baby grows. A retinal detachment is actually a separation of the nervous layer from the pigment layer of the retina.

Rhegmatogenous retinal detachment

A rhegma is a hole. A simple hole in the retina rarely causes symptoms and may be discovered during a routine eye test. Occasionally the ophthalmologist may decide not to treat the hole, and observe it instead over a period of time. According to Ghazi and Green (2001) this is because 'formed vitreous gel acts as a seal to retinal breaks and indirectly prevents retinal detachment'. A rhegmatogenous retinal detachment occurs when the retinal layers are detached from one another as the result of a tear, break or hole, allowing sub-retinal fluid to accumulate between the nervous and pigment layers.

There are several causes of rhegmatogenous retinal detachment:

Short-sightedness: A 'short sighted' person has a physiologically longer eye, and as a result, the retina is stretched more tightly across the back of the eye. In the myopic eye therefore there is a greater tendency for the layers of the retina to detach as a result of a tear. The incidence of myopia varies across populations, and with family hereditary factors, but Kanski (2007) states that myopia affects 10% of the population. He goes on to say that 40% of all retinal detachments occur in myopic eyes. Highly myopic people with prescriptions ranging from –5 to –20 are at an even greater risk of developing retinal detachment. Unfortunately high myopia is an inherited tendency and may be accompanied by a family history of retinal detachments. You can read a well-illustrated article on the subject of retinal detachments by Larkin (2006).

Cataract surgery: The Department of Health (2008) recognises that cataract surgery (in addition to myopia) is a predisposing factor for retinal detachment. They quantify it as causing a 0.7% increased risk of retinal detachment.

Ageing: Ageing makes a person increasingly susceptible to developing a retinal detachment. Riordan-Eva *et al.* (2003) state that syneresis (shrinking of the vitreous gel) affects 60% of people aged over 60. Shrinking of the vitreous is significant because it is attached to the retina at the pars plana of the ciliary body, at the optic disc and macula. As the 'shrinking vitreous' moves with rotational eye movements, sufficient 'pulling' forces may be generated to cause the retina to tear at an area where it is attached to the vitreous, for example at the optic disc margins, macula, along the main blood vessels – causing vitreous haemorrhage – and at the pars plana. Any further traction will cause the tear to increase. By the age of about 60 (Kanski, 1994) about 65% of the vitreous will have liquefied. Syneresis is the word used to describe the process by which the ageing vitreous gel contracts and fluid separates out. Photopsia is a symptom of these vitreous changes, and is described medically as flashing lights in the visual field.

Retinal tears are another cause of rhegmatogenous detachment and sometimes occur in a susceptible person in response to injury. Blunt trauma to the eye, for example from a football or a fist, may cause a retinal tear, as may a bang to the head as in an elderly person who falls.

Lattice degeneration affects 7% of the population (Riordan-Eva *et al.*, 2003). It is a type of retinal thinning that runs around the circumference of the eye from the ora serata and sometimes leads to full-thickness retinal holes developing at the lesions. It is a feature of ageing, but may develop earlier in myopic people. Kanski (1994) states that 40% of people with retinal detachments are noted to have lattice degeneration, particularly myopic people.

To do …

Find out what causes photopsia.

Ask a patient who has reported photopsia to describe it to you in their own words. Do keep listening to how patients express themselves non-medically, so that you develop a better understanding of what they are trying to tell you.

What is a **vitreous floater**? What causes them? Are they serious?

Is there anything you are looking to find in a patient's description of vitreous floaters that would alert you immediately to the possibility of an impending detachment?

You will find most of the answers to the above in *Optometry Today* (Kabat and Sowka's article on posterior vitreous detachment).

You may sometimes read in a patient's notes that they have posterior vitreous detachment (PVD). You can find out more about this at the *Good Hope* website.

To do ...

Can you find a definition for lattice degeneration?
What is (usually) the treatment for this?
How are myopic eyes affected?

Look for the answers to these questions in the article by Bruce available on the Optician Online website.

The treatments for rhegmatogenous retinal detachment are:

- laser to seal small tears
- cryothermy to lattice for small tears
- explant (plomb/encirclement)
- retinopexy insertion of gas
- silicone tamponade
- vitrectomy.

Macular hole

A macular hole is a tiny full-thickness retinal hole at the macula, occurring predominantly in women. It causes central visual distortion, and generally affects only one eye. If the hole is not treated it may lead to retinal detachment, but successful surgery can improve sight. Treatment is by vitrectomy, insertion of gas and posturing.

See the Patient UK website for an article by Willacy on macular holes.

Tractional retinal detachment

A rare cause of this type of detachment is retinopathy of prematurity (ROP). This condition used to be known as retrolental fibroplasia and it is linked to premature babies and the oxygen levels they receive in neonatal incubators to keep them alive. Abnormalities occur in the developing retinal blood vessels. Laser treatment may be needed to seal them and prevent retinal detachment. Today's treatments are effective in ensuring reasonable visual outcomes if they are carried out in time. However, if you work with adults, you may meet an older person who was born before the need to check the retinas of premature babies was understood, and before laser treatment was available. There is no cure at this stage. They may comment when you go to test their eyes that their poor vision is due to prematurity and being nursed in an incubator with high oxygen levels.

A lucid explanation of this condition is available on the Royal College of Ophthalmologists website.

Diabetic retinopathy may also cause a tractional retinal detachment. This is due to problems with the microvascular circulation of the retina. High blood sugar levels and raised blood pressure eventually lead to thickening and blockage of the microcirculation. Resultant damage to the basement membrane of the retina causes release of VEGF (vascular endothelial growth factor). This stimulates the growth of new, immature blood vessels growing forward from the retina into the vitreous. If these new blood vessels are left to bleed and leak into the vitreous, scar tissue can develop around them, which shrinks and can cause a tractional retinal detachment. Treatment of this condition is vitrectomy (removal of the vitreous), and a gas bubble may be inserted into the eye to hold the detached layers together. Direct laser treatment can be applied to the retina at the time of surgery.

Check out Birmingham University's MedWeb site to find out more about laser treatments to the diabetic eye, and many other aspects of diabetes for the general public and medical professionals.

Obviously good control of blood sugar levels and general health is likely to slow the development of this condition in people with type 1 diabetes. However, some unfortunate people whose type 2 diabetes is not discovered promptly may present with quite severe diabetic retinopathy on diagnosis. Treatment is by laser applied specifically to the problem with new vessels and the area in which they occur. If bleeding within the vitreous has resulted in visual loss, vitrectomy and laser treatment may improve the person's vision a little.

Exudative retinal detachment

Exudative detachments are very rare. They arise from fluid accumulating under the retina due to tumours and inflammation. Treatment is directed to the underlying cause.

Nursing management of a patient with retinal detachment

To do ...

List as many symptoms of retinal detachment as you can find.

If a patient is booked into an ophthalmic accident and emergency department with suspected retinal detachment, ophthalmic nurses or professionals allied to medicine (PAMs) would generally be expected to obtain and accurately document:

- a history of the patient's presenting ocular/visual symptoms.
- a history of the patient's past ocular diseases and conditions.
- a family history of eye problems.
- a relevant social history including occupation.
- a summary of the patient's current past and current general health.
- a history of current medications for ocular and general health.
- a history of any allergies/adverse reactions to treatments.
- a note of any areas of particular concern.

They would also:

- test and accurately record visual acuity
- measure and record intraocular pressure
- make a preliminary slit lamp examination of the anterior chamber
- check for a relative afferent pupil defect
- check for red reflex.

These have been summarised from the National Occupational Standards and relate directly to Health and well-being HWB6 assessment and treatment planning level 3. See the *Association of Health Professionals in Ophthalmology* website.

To do ...

Would you expect to find any deviations from normal in the above findings?

Discuss your thoughts with your mentor.

Preoperative care

This is likely to include:

- dilating both pupils for retinal examination on medical prescription or using relevant departmental protocol
- providing appropriate education for patient and relatives and continuing to answer any questions arising over the treatment period
- arranging preoperative ward admission (if required)
- mobility issues – whether at home or in hospital awaiting surgery, the patient and the people caring for him or her need to know if they will be allowed to walk around freely or whether there are limits to their activities; advise the patient regarding appropriate exercise and diet during any periods of limited mobility.

Sometimes patients are required to rest preoperatively in a prescribed position. Check with the ophthalmologist to find out whether this is necessary. Positioning normally involves resting with the retinal hole in the lowest possible position (e.g. head to the affected side if the hole is medial or lateral). Some patients with inferior holes are required to sit, but those with holes in the superior position may have to rest with their head lower than the rest of their body. The reason for this is to use gravity to allow the vitreous to rest on top of the hole, lessening the chances of the area of detachment increasing. Positioning prior to surgery is highly relevant for patients with superior retinal detachments, where the macula is still 'on' (attached to the underlying layers of the retina), and it is important to keep it 'on'. Detachment surgery continues to improve, but the prognosis for clear central vision is poorer if the macula is 'off' (detached from the underlying layers of the retina).

Intraoperative care

Surgery may take place under local or general anaesthesia according to the patient's general health and the type of surgery being undertaken. Normally for cryothermy, application of a plomb or silicone band general anaesthesia would be used, as there is a lot of pulling on the external ocular muscles.

From the scrub person's point of view, all retinal surgery is very taxing, as the theatre is in semi-darkness to facilitate the surgeon's intraoperative view through the lens of the indirect ophthalmoscope or operating microscope. The anaesthetist will use one of the theatre 'spot' lamps to check the patient's general condition, but management of the surgical instruments on the trolley can be difficult in between 'lights on' and 'lights off' at the surgeon's behest. This also makes what is happening very difficult for the rest of the staff to observe and anticipate.

Cryothermy

Cryothermy may be used to freeze the detached retinal layers together temporarily. This process produces scar tissue that forms a more permanent bond between the layers after about 2 weeks. It is only suitable for tears that are too large for laser treatment, and very small areas of detachment.

Plomb

A plomb (sometimes called a scleral buckle) is a piece of silicone material that is sewn to the outside of a patient's eye (but underneath the conjunctiva) in order to produce an indentation over an area of retinal detachment. Sub-retinal fluid is withdrawn using a needle and cryothermy is applied to the outside of the eye to produce a sterile reaction to 'stick' the areas of the retina together. Success in this approach to surgery is dependent on the plomb being correctly placed over the hole.

Silicone band

This is sometimes referred to as an 'encirclement' or 'strap'. A silicone band is threaded under the four rectus muscles and tightened around the eye. It was used for patients with multiple retinal tears, a lot of vitreous traction or retinal tears beyond the equator of the eye. It can be painful for some time both immediately post surgery and following discharge, because of the extent to which the intraocular muscles are handled and the tightness of the band. Theatre staff must check that effective analgesia and anti-emetics are prescribed for the immediate postoperative period before handing over their patient.

For the three surgical approaches above, the surgeon will make use of an indirect ophthalmoscope and hand held lens to visualise the retina.

Vitrectomy and intravitreal gas (pneumatic retinopexy) or silicone oil

This is an increasingly popular approach to retinal detachment, because operating from within the eye has several advantages:

- the surgeon can remove any haemorrhage or scar tissue by posterior vitrectomy
- insertion of gas or oil – pneumatic retinopexy holds the detached area of retina in place by applying pressure within the eye (it is significantly less painful post surgery)
- cryothermy or laser are used to seal the retinal hole.

The procedures are conducive to local anaesthesia and there is the possibility of day surgery, provided that the patient will not be alone and has adequate pain control supplied for use at home.

Vitrectomy procedures are often combined with cataract surgery because vitrectomy may cause cataract development.

To do ...

Make a list of other retinal disorders treated by vitrectomy.

What are the advantages of using intravitreal silicone oil instead of gas?

What are the problems with measuring the biometry of a silicone oil-filled eye, and how may such problems be avoided?

Postoperative care following retinal surgery

Fresh advice must be sought from the surgeon regarding postoperative positioning if a gas bubble has been inserted into the vitreous. This is because patients must be helped into position so that the gas bubble floats up to support the layer of detached retina in position while adhesion takes place. They will be required to maintain the prescribed position for most of the time – day and night – for up to 3 weeks after surgery, as the gas bubble is gradually absorbed. They should never lie on their back because the gas bubble will settle behind their iris and lens, reducing the drainage angle, which is likely to give rise to symptoms of an acute secondary glaucoma. It is helpful to patients who must be positioned to spend the postoperative night in hospital where they can be shown how to position properly while both waking and sleeping, how to get comfortable, and how to maintain the position. It is useful and reassuring if there is a nursing contact they can ring on discharge if they have any problems or questions that need answering.

If the patient needs to position face-down following macular hole surgery, remember at the preoperative interview to suggest that they wear comfortable clothing, without tight collars or buttons down the front. Pillows, rolled towels and blankets should be used to assist the patient in maintaining the prescribed position. Remember that they will need plenty of practical advice and emotional support during this period.

There is no immediate, obvious improvement in vision while a gas bubble is present, and health professionals should be careful not to raise patients' expectations of visual improvement post surgery.

If a silicone band has been applied to the eye, anterior segment ischaemia is a rare postoperative complication due to venous compression by the plomb or band.

Excessive pain in the immediate postoperative period is a significant symptom, which needs to be reported promptly.

Following retinal surgery, patients will need to bathe their eyelids clean as necessary, using normal saline or cool, boiled water. If surgery involved the use of a plomb or encirclement surgery, a clear, extremely sticky exudate is produced as part of the healing process, which dries like a hard 'glue' and can cause a lot of discomfort, particularly on waking, as the eyelashes and lids are often 'glued' together. If the patient gently applies a 'sloppy wet' gauze swab to the eyelids for several minutes, the eye will begin to open.

Considerable swelling of the eyelids can be expected in the normal progress of recovery following the application of a plomb or an encirclement, particularly following cryothermy. The swelling is sometimes worse on day two and three, and may – on waking – be noted to have spread to the unoperated eye, particularly when the patient is being positioned on the unoperated side. Patients get alarmed by this. Cold compresses are helpful for relieving any swelling and aching around the operated eye. A transparent cartella shield may be worn at night for the first week following surgery to avoid accidental damage during the night.

Discharge advice

Good preoperative preparation will help to prevent patients experiencing most difficulties on discharge.

Positioning

The patient's plans to cope with their limited activities postoperatively should be discussed with them as soon as possible. This needs to include planning for meals and shopping for food. Relatives and friends may need to assist. Microwaveable meals may be easier and quicker to prepare for someone who lives alone. Suitable activities also need to be planned to fill their leisure time, and might include listening to the radio or 'talking books'. For patients required to keep their 'head down', large-print books, playing cards or board games may be useful. Regular visitors can be very helpful too. Short car journeys (as a passenger!) make visits to relatives and friends' homes possible if the prescribed head position can be maintained in the car and on arrival. Maintaining the prescribed position is a major contributor to the success of the eye surgery. Equipment to help with positioning while sitting at home (such as a small adjustable table and pillow to rest the head) on will need to be considered.

Eye care

You will need to discuss anticipated swelling and discomfort, eye bathing if necessary, eye-drop instillation, pain relief and a telephone contact just in case the patient has any concerns or needs further advice. This verbal guidance should be backed up with a printed patient guide on the condition. Make sure that the patient can instil their eye-drops and has an adequate supply of prescribed medications. An outpatient follow-up appointment must be booked, and should include transport arrangements if necessary.

Air travel

This is not permitted for patients who have had intravitreal gas inserted, as the slightly lower air pressure in the cabin during flight will cause the gas to expand and the intraocular pressure to rise. The gas is absorbed naturally within a few weeks following insertion.

To do ...

What different ideas have you tried to help patients with posturing?

How does the ophthalmologist know whether the patient has been carrying out the positioning as instructed? (You may need to ask an ophthalmologist!)

Other retinal problems

Commotio retinae

This condition often follows a sport-related blunt injury to the eye of a child or young adult. It may be associated with a hyphaema. The injury causes a disruption and fragmentation of the photoreceptor segments of the retina and the retinal pigment epithelium (Meyer *et al.*, 2003). On examination, the retina, particularly at the periphery, looks milky white with oedema. Vision is likely to be disturbed for weeks or months later. There is no treatment, and the condition normally resolves spontaneously.

To do ...

What further problems might commotio lead to?

Retinitis pigmentosa

This term refers to a group of inherited retinal dystrophies with a range of severity and symptoms. As there is no current recognised treatment, genetic counselling and social support are the primary means of management. However, these people may have some vision, which it is important to preserve, and may be seen in the eye department for cataract surgery, for example. Possible future treatments may include gene therapy and the transplantation of healthy retinal cells.

You can find additional information at the EyeHelp website.

Diabetic eye disease

Diabetic retinopathy is the leading cause of blindness in the working aged population of the UK (Department of Health, 2008). Helping to prevent some cases of type 2 diabetes through greater public awareness about good nutrition and exercise is of primary importance, as is screening for diabetes and careful monitoring of all people with diabetes. Effective annual screening programmes are available to people with diabetes via selected optometrists' practices that now include digital colour photographs of the retina through dilated pupils.

People with type 1 diabetes are likely to develop changes to their microvascular retinal circulation within 20 years of onset. Good glycaemic control will slow these inevitable changes, and prophylactic laser treatments.

Morello (2007) states that 'retinopathy is already present at the time of diagnosis in 20% of people with type 2 diabetes'. This is due to the insidious nature of type 2 diabetes – of this 20%, a few may attend as ophthalmic emergencies with the presenting symptom of deteriorating vision.

Over the last 40 years, much of the blindness associated with diabetes has been prevented by the use of superior insulin, accurate blood sugar monitoring and treatment with an ophthalmic laser. More recently anti-VEGF (vascular endothelial growth factor) treatments have been used in the event that laser treatment fails to control the eye condition.

Points to consider

Pupil dilatation

People with diabetes will need regular photographs to record the progression of any retinal changes. For these and laser treatments, good wide pupil dilatation is essential, and drops will be either individually prescribed or instilled by nurses under local protocols. Generally a combination of different types of eye-drops is used, usually a cycloplegic and sympathomimetic as the different actions of each eye-drop will enhance the effects of the other.

 Make sure that you are aware of potential side effects when using these eye-drops, as people with diabetes may also have a range of other health problems.

 Nurse prescribers should be aware that research by Weiss *et al.* (1995) on 127 people with diabetes indicated that phenylephrine 2.5% used in combination with a mydriatic showed no statistically significant difference in the dilatation achieved compared to a 10% solution used alone in the fellow eye. They recommend the use of the 2.5% solution for this patient group who have a higher than average prevalence of vascular disease and autonomic dysfunction.

 People with diabetes often drive to their appointments so that they can get back to work immediately. A binocular visual acuity of 6/9 is required for UK driving (Driver and Vehicle Licensing Agency, 2006). Jude *et al.* (1998) noted a reduction in binocular visual acuity (BVA) post dilatation which, with the addition of glare, caused visual acuity to drop further, even when using sunglasses. They concluded that patients need to be warned not to drive post dilatation. Murgatroyd *et al.* (2006) advised that retinal screeners need to have clear guidelines with which to advise patients regarding driving safety.

Time management

Remember that people who have had diabetes since childhood have attended many, many medical appointments, and are anxious to get on with their lives. In some health areas Joint Retinal Clinics run with physicians and ophthalmologists attending have reduced the need for some attendances, as has the advent of portable laser machines, which can be taken to these clinics to laser potentially leaky retinal vessels as soon as possible.

Laser safety

Remember the necessity for wearing the correct goggles whenever you are present during laser treatments. A laser safety officer must instruct and update you regularly on safe practice in your department. Goggles suitable for one type of laser are unsuitable for another. Make sure that the correct goggles are stored with each machine, and do not migrate from one laser room to another. Warning lights outside the doors of treatment areas must be switched on for the duration of treatments.

Pigmented retinal naevi

Make a web search for more information on this. The Digital Reference of Ophthalmology has some other interesting retinal areas you can explore too. You could also look at the Eye Cancer Network, where you can find information about choroidal melanoma.

Retinal vein occlusion

A retinal vein occlusion is caused by a tiny blood clot either in the central retinal vein or one of its smaller tributaries. Generally they occur in people over the age of 50. According to the Royal College of Ophthalmologists guidelines (2009), hypertension, hyperlipidaemia, diabetes mellitus and glaucoma are the main predisposing factors for this condition, which results in oedema at the optic disc, dilated retinal veins and deep and superficial haemorrhages.

The patient presents with painless mild to severe loss of vision in the affected eye, which looks normal. On presentation with a sudden loss of vision, the nurse should check blood pressure and blood glucose (or urinalysis). A relative afferent pupillary defect (RAPD) may be present. Ring the ophthalmologist with these results, and carry out any further instructions.

There is no effective treatment for this condition. When the diagnosis is confirmed, the ophthalmologist will refer the patient urgently to the physician. Outpatient follow-up will be at 3 months, when photocoagulation will be required if a quadrant or more of the retina was involved to prevent neovascularisation (the growth of abnormal new blood vessels) as this could lead to neovascular glaucoma. This neovascular glaucoma is caused by the abnormal blood vessels growing forward on to the iris, through the pupil and into the drainage angle, gradually blocking the aqueous outflow. Following laser treatment the patient is usually reviewed at least at 6-monthly intervals for 2 years.

Check the Good Hope Hospital website for more information about retinal vein occlusion and watch the little movie which shows how this condition can lead to rubeotic glaucoma, and see how this is treated. It is good for you to read about it and you may consider using it for patients. There are even patient leaflets you can download if you do not have any.

Retinal artery occlusion

This presents rather like retinal vein occlusion but the loss of vision when the central retinal artery is involved is very sudden and severe, generally reduced to counting fingers or hand movements. This painless condition presents in a similar way to venous occlusion inasmuch as the eye looks 'normal' in appearance. Because the differentiation between artery occlusion and vein occlusion can only be definitely made on ophthalmoscopy, if you do not have recognised competency, then both the venous occlusion and artery occlusion must be treated as emergency sudden painless loss of vision. Check blood pressure and blood glucose (or urinalysis). Check for a relative afferent pupillary defect. Ring the ophthalmologist with the results, and carry out any instructions you are given. Immediate treatment is normally instituted if the blockage has occurred within 'a few hours' (Kanski, 2007). Beyond this time, it is unlikely that vision will improve, but in fact treatment for this condition is rarely successful.

The main predisposing factors of this condition are cigarette smoking, cardiovascular disease, hypertension, carotid artery disease and hyperlipidaemia. The actual material blocking the artery may be derived from deposits on damaged heart valves, or may be thrombotic or from atheroma of the carotid artery.

Graham and Ebrahim (2007) list current possible treatments for retinal artery occlusion as:

- intraocular pressure reduction, possibly using intravenous acetazolamide (500 mg) and/or intraocular pressure-reducing eye-drops
- anterior chamber paracentesis (local anaesthetic drops are applied to the eye; a 30 gauge needle is attached to an insulin syringe and used to withdraw about 0.01–0.02 mL of aqueous fluid; antibiotic cover may be given post procedure)
- fibrinolysis with urokinase (has been used, but controversial with major side effects).

 When you ring the ophthalmologist, you could enquire whether they would like the following two simple treatments commenced while the patient waits for their examination:

Massage: This is done by applying direct gentle digital pressure to the eye over an eyepad or some swabs for 15 seconds, then releasing it. This is repeated several times and may gently push the blockage further through the arterial system to improve the circulation to the retina.

Breathing in and out of a paper bag. This increases carbon dioxide levels and promotes vasodi-latation to enable the tiny clot to move to a less damaging area.

In addition to the above, the ophthalmologist will normally commence aspirin therapy and make an urgent medical referral for the management of the patient's overall condition. Field and Tillotson (2008) comment that it is unwise to over-reassure the patient regarding the sight loss, but they do need the assurance that everything possible was done to try to save their sight. Given the predisposing causes for this condition, you might personally reflect that even if the patient's sight was not saved, at least their life expectancy may be considerably extended.

 Further information is available at the *Handbook of Ocular Disease Management* and more academic detail is given in an article by Law (2007) at *eMedicine.*

References and further reading

Bruce, A., O'Day, J., McKay, J., *et al.* (2007). Lattice degeneration.
Available at: www.opticianonline.net/assets/getAsset.aspx?ItemID = 2457 (last accessed August 2009).

Department of Health (2008). Diabetic Retinopathy Screening Statement. Available at:
http://www.dh.gov.uk/en/Publicationsandstatistics/Publications/PublicationsPolicyAndGuidance/DH_083895
(last accessed August 2009).

Driver and Vehicle Licensing Agency (2006). *Visual Disorders, Medical Rules.* London: DVLA.

Field, D. and Tillotson, J. (2008). *Eye Emergencies: The practitioner's guide.* Keswick: M&K Update.

Ghazi, N. and Green, W. (2002). Pathology and pathogenesis of retinal detachment. *Eye*, 16, 411–21.

Graham, R. and Ebrahim, S. (2007). Central Retinal Artery Occlusion.
Available at: http://www.emedicine.com/OPH/topic387.htm (last accessed August 2009).

Jude, E., Ryan, B., O'Leary, B., Gibson, J. and Dodson, P. (1998). Pupillary dilatation and driving in diabetic patients.
Diabetic Medicine: Journal of the British Diabetic Association, 15(2), 143–47.

Kabat, A. and Sowka, J. (2001). A clinician's guide to flashes and floaters. *Optometry Today*, 23, 3–37.
Available at: www.optometry.co.uk/articles/docs/640c1a5b606a7d89320511ca29ccc288_kabat20010323.pdf
(last accessed August 2009).

Kanski, J. (1994). *Clinical Ophthalmology*, 4th edn. Oxford: Butterworth Heinemann.

Kanski, J. (2007). *Clinical Ophthalmology*, 7th edn. Oxford: Butterworth Heinemann.

Larkin, G. (2006). Retinal detachment. Available at: http://www.emedicine.com/emerg/topic504.htm
(last accessed August 2009). Click on 'multimedia' at the right of the screen to find the pictures.

Law, J. (2007). Branch retinal artery occlusion. Available at: http://www.emedicine.com/OPH/topic385.htm
(last accessed August 2009).

Marsden, J. (2004). Implications of and treatment options for retinal detachment. *Nursing Times*, 100(37), 44–47.

Meyer, C., Rodrigues, E. and Mennel, S. (2003). Acute como retinas determined by cross sectional optical coherence
tomography. *European Journal of Ophthalmology*, 13, 816–18.

Morello, C. (2007). Etiology and natural history of diabetic retinopathy: an overview. *American Journal of Health-System
Pharmacy*, 64, S3–S7.

Murgatroyd, H., MacEwen, C. and Leese, G. (2006). Patients' attitudes towards mydriasis for diabetic eye disease
screening. *Scottish Medical Journal*, 51(4), 35–37.

Riordan-Eva, P., Whitcher, J., Vaughan, D. and Asbury, T. (2003). *General Ophthalmology.* London: McGraw Hill.

Royal College of Ophthalmologists (2009). *Retinal Vein Occlusion – Interim Guidelines.* London: Royal College of
Ophthalmologists.

Waterman, H., Harker, R., MacDonald, H., McLaughlan, R. and Waterman, C. (2005). Advancing ophthalmic nursing
practice through action research. *Journal of Advanced Nursing*, 52(3), 281–90. (This paper reports an action research
project that promoted posturing face down following macular hole surgery and aimed to enhance patient outcomes.)

Weiss, J., Weiss, J. and Greenfield, D. (1995). The effects of phenylephrine 2.5% versus phenylephrine 10% on
pupillary dilation in patients with diabetes. *Retina*, 15(2), 130–33.

Willacy, H. (2007). Macular holes. Available at: http://www.patient.co.uk/showdoc/40002429/ (last accessed August 2009).

Useful web resources

Association of Health Professionals in Ophthalmology
http://www.ahpo.org/
You will find the National Occupational Standards here.

Digital Reference of Ophthalmology
http://dro.hs.columbia.edu/
For more information on vitreous and retina.

eMedicine from webMD
http://emedicine.medscape.com/
*For articles by Graham on central retinal artery occlusion, Larkin on retinal detachment (click on Multimedia at the right of
the screen to find the pictures) and Law on branch retinal artery occlusion.*

Eye Cancer Network
http://www.eyecancer.com/
Look for information on choroidal nevus.

EyeHelp.co.uk
http://www.eyehelp.co.uk/
Retinitis pigmentosa information.

Good Hope Hospital
http://www.goodhope.org.uk/

Handbook of Ocular Disease Management
http://www.revoptom.com/HANDBOOK/default.htm
Search for central retinal artery occlusion, retinal vein occlusion and commotio retinae.

MedWeb at the University of Birmingham
http://medweb.bham.ac.uk/easdec/
Hosts to the European Association for the Study of Diabetic Eye Complications (EASDEC).

Optician Online
http://www.opticianonline.net/Home/Default.aspx
Look for the article by Bruce, O'Day and McKay on lattice degeneration.

Optometry Today
http://www.optometry.co.uk/.

Patient UK
http://www.patient.co.uk/
Willacy has written an article on macular holes.

Review of Optometry
http://www.revoptom.com/
Information on vitreous and retina.

Royal College of Ophthalmologists
http://www.rcophth.ac.uk/
Search retinopathy of prematurity, and retinal vein occlusion.

SELF TEST answers on page 206

1. Name two possible causes of retinal tears.

2. Name two treatment approaches to rhegmatogenous retinal detachment.

3. Premature babies in oxygenated incubators may develop what?

4. Does diabetic retinopathy affect people with type 1 or type 2 diabetes?

5. Why may it be necessary to 'position' a patient with a superior retinal detachment?

6. Why might the application of a silicone encircling band be particularly painful postoperatively?

7. What does commotio retinae result from?

8. What type of glaucoma may follow a retinal vein occlusion?

9. Name two predisposing factors to retinal artery occlusion.

Chapter 12

Age-related macular degeneration

Dorothy Field and Mandy Macfarlane

On completion of this topic you will:

- understand what macular degeneration is
- know about the early detection and treatment of different types of degeneration
- be aware of the available diagnostic tests and investigations
- appreciate the significance of offering health education and suggesting lifestyle changes to your client groups.

Background

The macula is contained within an area of the retina called the fundus. It is prone to age changes like all other structures of the human body. With ageing, cellular structures deteriorate and atrophy (waste away).

You may see the name of this condition abbreviated in patient records and in the media. It is commonly called AMD, but ARMD is sometimes used in older documentation. AMD is an eye condition that leads to a progressive loss of central vision. People generally retain their peripheral vision, but the ability to see well enough to recognise faces, drive and read is grossly compromised, often leading to anxiety and depression. Owen *et al.* (2003) pooled data from six studies in the UK and concluded that the prevalence of visual loss caused by AMD increased exponentially from the age of 70 to 85 years of age. The authors estimate that there are currently 214,000 people with visual impairment caused by AMD (suitable for registration). They expect this number to increase to 239,000 by the year 2011.

Factors that may contribute to the development of AMD

Genetic factors

These have been known for some years to influence the development of AMD (Antoniak *et al.*, 2008). Additionally, Baird *et al.* (2008) recently discovered an interaction between genetic factors, the environment the person lives in, and exposure to chronic infection, which may be involved in progression of the disease.

Smoking

Research by Cong *et al.* (2008) indicates that smoking, especially current smoking, was significantly associated with an increased risk of AMD and its subtypes.

Obesity

Connections between obesity and any increased risk of developing AMD are inconsistent. However, Johnson (2005) inferred that the mechanism by which obesity increased the rate of AMD development might be related to the physiological changes associated with increased weight gain, which include oxidative stress.

Race

Bressler *et al.* (2008) noted that white people were more likely than black people to have medium or large drusen, pigment abnormalities and advanced AMD. Their data suggests that black people may have a natural mechanism for protection against these changes in the fundus area.

Gender

Women have higher rates of AMD than men (Klein *et al.* 1992; Javitt *et al.* (2003). However, Feskanich *et al.* (2008) noted that current post menopausal hormone replacement (HRT) users had a 48% lower risk of neovascular AMD compared with those who had never used HRT. The risk of developing AMD was lowest for HRT users who had previously used oral contraceptives. There was a 26% lower risk of developing early AMD for parous women. The proportionately greater risk to women might in fact be attributable to their greater longevity.

Diet

Tan's (2008) population-based study demonstrated that dietary antioxidants reduced the risk of AMD.

Prolonged sun exposure

The effects of light exposure on the development of AMD are not satisfactorily proven. The difficulty of estimating light exposure in a large sample is a problem.

How AMD develops

As noted above, AMD is a condition that develops in mature people. Its causes, at a cellular level, are still not fully understood, but Zarbin (2004) provides a credible five-stage analysis which is summarised below:

1. AMD is linked to the ageing process and is multifactorial.

2. Oxidative stress (explained simply in an article by Rutherford (2007) on the Net Doctor website) results in damage to the retinal pigment epithelium and possibly secondarily to the choroidal blood flow.

3. Damage to the retinal pigment epithelium (see Fig. 2.8) leads to chronic inflammation within Bruch's membrane, which lies between the retinal pigment epithelium and the choroid.

4. Damage and inflammation in the choroidal circulation leads to the formation of an abnormal extracellular matrix that alters the diffusion of nutrients to the retina and retinal pigment epithelium, resulting in further retinal damage.

5. The abnormal extracellular matrix results in changes to the retinal circulation, resulting in atrophy and new blood vessel growth in the choroid.

This is, of course, just one theory among many, but all of them are similar. Friedman (2008) also points to the theory of impaired choroidal perfusion and the development of drusen (tiny yellow deposits lying beneath the retinal blood vessels, which can merge into larger masses) in the pathogenesis of AMD, and additionally highlights the increase in scleral rigidity which accompanies ageing and serves to impair choroidal perfusion.

Classification of AMD

AMD can be classified into two types:

dry AMD – this accounts for around 90% of the total number of people with AMD

wet AMD – this occurs in around 10% of people with AMD.

The way the AMD is classified will determine the treatment.

Symptoms of AMD

These include:

- metamorphosia (distortion in the central field where straight lines appear bent)
- subdued colour perception

- sudden reduction in central visual acuity; or

- gradual reduction leading eventually to a central scotoma (blind spot) that occurs as a result of scar tissue formation (this is obviously a sign rather than a symptom).

> The above is based on Haque (2000) and can be found on *Pharmacy Journal Online* website. Often the optometrist will already have noticed that the patient is developing this condition because the formation of increased drusen at the macular area is an early warning sign.

Nursing care and interventions for patients

Routes of referral to the fast track medical macular clinic can be:

direct: via a general practitioner or ophthalmic optometrist, or

indirect: via facsimile from a general practitioner or optometrist to the acute referral clinic/eye accident and emergency, or by self-referral over the telephone or by attending as a walk-in to the acute clinic or emergency department.

Having a comprehensive evidence-based knowledge of the symptoms of AMD is an essential requirement for any health professional responsible for receiving patient referrals from any of the above sources. It is of paramount importance that the pathway of investigation, treatment and ongoing management is initiated urgently as a narrow window of treatment opportunity may easily be missed, resulting in detrimental consequences to a patient's lifestyle, mental health and longevity.

New patient referral

It is important that the nurse gives clear explanations to the patient about the assessment process and its purpose. The visual assessment will form the baseline from which treatment is judged to be effective and therefore a high degree of accuracy and care should be taken with the measurements and the recording of them.

Tests and investigations for wet and dry AMD

On arrival the ophthalmic nurse may perform a range of initial visual assessments. This might include checks of:

- distance visual acuity in both eyes (logMAR chart)
- wavy lines or distortions (Amsler charts for both eyes)
- reading visual acuity (near-vision tests)
- colour vision monitoring (Ishihara's test)
- relative afferent pupillary defect (RAPD)

- dilation of the pupils (both eyes)
- visual acuity (Snellen, logMAR and near-vision tests).

These tests are used to establish a diagnosis in the case of both dry and wet forms of AMD and to form a baseline for subsequent comparison on each visit in the case of wet AMD. The levels of nursing input will vary greatly from one clinic to another and will largely depend on the leading clinician as to the number of technical skills a nurse may need to perform proficiently.

To do ...

Find out how this group of patients is assessed in your eye department.

Health and safety

Often it is a nurse who administers dilating drops to both eyes for the purpose of fundoscopy, either from written instructions by the doctor in the patient record or under the parameters of a patient group directive. Prior to administration it is important to ask patients whether they have any allergies, or are taking any medications, or have had any ophthalmic-related problems in the past. Patients should be instructed not to drive to their appointments because the mydriatic and cycloplegic effect of tropicamide cyclopentolate and phenylephrine interfere with the ability to focus and significantly blur the vision and cause photophobia. This may prohibit driving under the terms of many vehicle insurance policies, so the mode of transport to the patient's home should be verified prior to dilation. These measures should be in place routinely to ensure patient safety and to fulfil our duty of care to the patient and our professional accountability in line with the code of the Nursing and Midwifery Council (NMC, 2008).

Examination by the clinician usually includes an intraocular pressure check and retinal fundoscopy. Investigations are ordered to confirm or establish a diagnosis and will provide a baseline for future comparisons. Most commonly, optical coherence tomography (OCT) and a fundus fluorescein angiography are conducted, but an indocyanine green angiography is requested if an occult (choroidal) lesion is suspected. A photographer, technician or nurse with additional skills may perform the imaging process.

Angiography

On examination of the retina the ophthalmologist may detect drusen and a raised lesion at the macula. Exudates may be present but often a fluorescein angiogram is required to confirm this. It involves an intravenous injection of fluorescein dye and a series of photographs that chart the progress of the dye as it flows through the retinal blood vessels. Identification of choroidal neovascularisation (CNV) on the fluorescein angiogram is made by studying the leakage pattern on different stages of the images. Comparing earlier images with the later ones enables leakage assessment. A diagnosis of classic or occult wet AMD is based on the time taken for any leakages to show up in the pictures and the areas involved. Indocyanine green is sometimes used instead of fluorescein as it is said to provide superior imaging of the choroidal circulation.

A trained nurse may undertake the administration of intravenous substances for the purpose of angiography. The nurse must be present throughout the procedure because, albeit rarely, anaphylaxis may occur; the patient may also experience a number of other less serious side effects.

We have a duty of care to ensure patients are fully informed and given information in a format appropriate to aid their comprehension. Due to nursing accountability, full consent should be sought from the patient for these invasive procedures using the appropriate documentation. The patient should be carefully monitored during and after administration and a set period of time should pass before the patient is allowed to leave the department. Due to the rare but significant serious risks to a patient's health, it is recommended that nurses should have training and an annual update in intermediate life support and anaphylaxis management.

Optical coherence tomography (OCT)

This is being increasingly used to monitor the condition of the macula because it is non-invasive and can identify intraretinal, sub-retinal or sub-retinal pigment epithelium fluid. You can find out more about this from Mann (2007).

To do ...

Familiarise yourself with the above imaging techniques in practice, as you may in the future be involved with fast-track macular disease clinics and with fluorescein and indocyanine green angiography.

Wet (advanced) AMD

Fortunately only about one in ten patients is diagnosed with wet AMD. All people who have the wet form had the dry type first – whether they were aware of this or not – hence the term advanced macular degeneration. The onset is more acute, often with a rapid decrease in central visual acuity within a few days or weeks, which causes the person to seek treatment. The process begins with the formation of drusen at Bruch's membrane, which weakens the retinal pigment epithelium and then allows choroidal neovascularisation (the development of new, immature blood vessels from the choroid into the sub-retinal or sub-retinal pigment epithelium space). These new vessels exude fluids and they bleed, resulting in severe visual loss. Eventually this causes a disciform scar, at which point the person will be said to have 'end-stage' AMD.

As with all types of sudden-onset visual disturbance, obtaining assessment, diagnosis and treatment at the earliest opportunity is best for preservation of sight and prognosis. It is believed that genetic and environmental factors play a significant role in the development of both types of AMD. The value of routine eye tests by an optometrist cannot be over-emphasised for helping to identify early the potential for AMD before the person becomes symptomatic. Patients with AMD may be given Amsler charts to take home to self-monitor any changes so that further treatment may be sought early.

Treatments

Treatments continue to development rapidly. The treatments below were current at the time of writing.

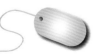 The National Institute for Clinical Excellence (NICE, 2008) has published revised guidelines on the use of ranibizumab (Lucentis™) and pegaptanib (Macugen™) in August 2008.

The NICE (2008) guidelines were required to settle disputes over the most effective treatment for wet AMD with the availability of new anti-VEGF (vascular endothelial growth factor) drugs. Within these guidelines, NICE stipulated that it does not currently recommend pegaptanib as a treatment for wet AMD. To qualify for treatment with ranibizumab, the following conditions must obtain for the affected eye:

- visual acuity must be between 6/12 and 6/9
- there should be no permanent damage to the fovea
- the lesion should be no more than 12 disc areas equivalent at its greatest linear dimension
- there must be evidence of disease progression either from fluorescein angiogram or a recent drop in visual acuity; and
- the manufacturer must meet the cost of ranibizumab beyond 14 injections.

In order for treatment to be continued, improvement in the eye condition must be maintained. It should be discontinued if the visual acuity continues to fall or anatomical changes in the retina indicate inadequate response to the treatment. At the time of writing, the NICE guidelines (2008) estimated the cost of ranibizumab injections alone to be about £10,700 to £18,300 over 2 years, and 26,000 new cases are expected per year.

As NICE has only authorised the use of ranibizumab, the issue being raised by some clinicians is why it is that – in the event of treatment failure – one of the two alternative treatments (pegaptanib or 'off label' products bevacizumab or Avastin™) cannot be tried.

Combination therapy

A large scale randomised controlled study in Europe known as 'Mont Blanc' is currently comparing the effectiveness of a combination treatment with verteporfin (Visudyne™) and ranibizumab (Lucentis™) compared with ranibizumab alone. The rationale behind this is that it offers the possibility of fewer treatments, thus lessening the risk of patients developing systemic side effects.

Common symptoms experienced by patients receiving ranibizumab injections are:

- subconjunctival haemorrhage for 2–48 hrs following injection (this is normal)
- 'black bubbles' in the visual field of the treated eye (commonly seen immediately after the injection) that may last up to 1 week, getting gradually smaller; these air bubbles are from the injection itself into the vitreous
- mild discomfort or grittiness for 2–48 hours (the eye should not be painful).

 Symptoms of particular concern following ranibizumab injection include:

- moderate or severe eye pain (possible endophthalmitis)
- sudden visual deterioration
- floaters and/or flashing lights.

In the event of any of these symptoms occurring, patients should use the telephone number they have been given to make urgent contact.

Prognosis

As a general guideline, patients should be advised during consultations that 30 % of those receiving a course of ranibizumab injections will see some improvement in vision, and that 90 % will achieve stable vision. How long these improvements might last for is unclear, but large studies are currently taking place.

The media has reported widely about the availability and positive effect on sight that intravitreal injection with either ranibizumab or bevacizumab can have. Patients may attend the medical macular clinic with preconceived expectations about a treatment that will 'cure' their eye problem. Not all of them will be treatable; intravitreal injections may only help reduce the impact of the neovascular (wet) AMD. However, Kaiser (2008) is optimistic, and states that clinical evidence to date shows statistically significant increases in the mean number of letters gained initially on logMAR testing.

The American Academy of Ophthalmology (Scott *et al.*, 2008) examined the evidence currently available for anti-VEGF drugs. They found reliable evidence that ranibizumab is an effective treatment for wet AMD for up to 2 years. Treatment does not, however, shrink the total size of the initial lesion.

 The University of Illinois' website **The Eye Digest** states that 'Lucentis™ clears the smoke (reduces leakage from CNV) and prevents the fire from spreading (halts the progression of CNV), but leaves the fire still burning (underlying disease process driving CNV is still active)'.

Treatment may therefore 'buy time' for patients to continue with their lives and remain independent. At no time should they be offered any hope that the injections are a 'cure all' due to the unpredictable nature of the disease process. It seems clinicians are reluctant to broach the subject of the likely outcome of wet AMD in the long term. Shielding patients from the realities of the condition may inadvertently hinder those who wish to plan ahead for a time when their vision levels may become significantly disabling. As the Eye Digest website puts it, most patients will continue to lose vision, albeit at a slower rate.

Photodynamic therapy (PDT)

 The evidence-based resource **Bandolier** (which reviews evidence-based health studies) concludes that PDT remains a cost effective treatment for people with milder forms of wet AMD, stating that it is a useful earlier form of treatment and remains reasonable value for money.

This treatment for wet AMD uses an intravenous injection of verteporfin (Visudyne™). It is picked up by the lipoproteins in the blood and taken up specifically by the abnormal retinal blood vessels. The verteporfin is activated by light and an ophthalmic laser is used to destroy and seal the abnormal retinal vessels. Not only is the verteporfin significantly expensive, but the patient and ophthalmologist require expert nursing support. Key nursing responsibilities are patient care, intravenous cannulation, monitoring and timing of the drug infusions, and continuous monitoring of the injection site.

Dry AMD

Cells at the macula atrophy but they do not release exudates. On fundoscopy (examination of the fundus), drusen (yellow deposits of waste products from the photoreceptors of the retina) are observed, as well as macular thinning and pigmentary disturbance due to the localised loss of retinal pigment epithelium (Wormald *et al.*, 2007). 'Hard' drusen are associated with dry AMD, and 'soft' drusen with wet AMD.

Treatment

Sadly, for people with dry AMD there is currently no treatment that retards the disease process. Fortunately its onset and progression are relatively slow and a reasonable level of visual acuity is usually maintained for longer compared with that of wet AMD. In the meantime, there is no harm in encouraging people to adopt some health strategies in the hope of slowing the progression of the disease.

 The **Royal National Institute for the Blind** (RNIB) suggests measures aimed at improving the general health, such as:

- stopping smoking
- reducing exposure to ultraviolet light and sunlight by using good quality sunglasses and a shady hat

- eating plenty of fruit and vegetables and foods rich in omega-3 fats (oily fish, omega-3-enriched eggs, green leafy vegetables, nuts, seed-enriched breads and rolls).

Further general health advice may include lowering blood cholesterol levels and good management of hypertension.

Diet

The AREDS study (Age-Related Eye Disease Research Group, 2001) showed that dietary supplements of antioxidant vitamins and zinc were associated with lower rates of the development of an AMD event or loss of visual acuity over 5 years. However, the results were dependent on how far the disease had already progressed prior to commencing the supplements. A Cochrane Review of published research by Evans (2006) on the effects of antioxidant vitamin or mineral supplements alone or in combination in the progression of AMD failed to establish a firm opinion on their utility. The review concluded that these supplements may cause a modest delay in the progression of the disease, but pointed out that there are harmful effects in the long term with such high doses, particularly in smokers or people with vascular disease. It recommended instead following a healthy diet that includes a variety of fresh fruit and vegetables, but pointed out that eating like this would make it difficult to consume the amounts of antioxidants and zinc prescribed in the trials. Evans (2006) also comments that the role of lutein and zeaxanthin is still unclear. Indirectly, this review does support the advice from RNIB regarding a healthy diet, so health professionals should encourage patients to adopt one. Rein *et al.* (2007) demonstrated the cost-effectiveness of vitamin therapy in people aged 50 years and above who were already diagnosed with AMD, with the caveat that beta-carotene should not be given to patients who smoke because the combination has been associated with the development of lung cancer.

Innovative developments

Research in improving the vision of people with dry AMD is ongoing and includes *implantation of intraocular lenses* for visually impaired people. These lenses are either miniature telescopes or a combination of individual lenses. The procedure is similar to a cataract operation, except that the special lenses are implanted. They divert images from the diseased macular to a healthy area of the retina. Patients require considerable visual rehabilitation postoperatively in order to gain the optical benefits. NICE has provided guidance on this procedure but points out that just because they have written interventional guidance does not mean NHS funding will be available for this procedure; such decisions must be taken by local primary care and hospital trusts based on whether they consider that this would constitute value for money.

A further trial, in the USA, involves *injecting human embryonic stem cells* into the diseased retina to regenerate retinal pigment epithelium cells. Similar experimental work is now being carried out at Moorfields hospital (MacLaren and Pearson, 2007).

Macular translocation

This is a surgical procedure that involves the deliberate detachment of the retina, with subsequent repositioning of the macula to a new location. Da Cruz (2007) records the use of this procedure to treat wet AMD. Such surgery can restore vision because it moves the retina away from the abnormal underlying vessels. It does however have major drawbacks in that the surgery is long and complicated and involves two operations. Significant post-surgical complications have been recorded, and as such this is never likely to become a mainstream treatment option.

To do ...

To get a feel for how AMD visual loss presents, try this:

- Start in a sitting position in a familiar room in good light.
- With your fingers, hold two small discs (or one-pence coins) by their edges at 6 o'clock.
- Hold each disc at their bottom edge between the thumb and forefinger.
- Continuing to hold the discs at their bottom edge, move them at eyelash distance directly over the centre of vision of each eye.
- Looking straight ahead only, move your head slowly around.
- Carefully stand up and attempt to navigate your way around the room.

Write down your thoughts and feelings about your experience.

Think about navigating through unfamiliar surroundings and performing everyday tasks such as going to the shops, choosing products and handling money.

Would you feel safe walking along the pavement among traffic or strangers?

How would you identify the items you needed to buy?

Would you know if you gave the right money and received the correct change?

Could you operate a cash machine and tell what denomination the notes were?

How would you prepare vegetables, use your oven or hob to cook, or know where the cup is when pouring boiling water or when the cup is nearly full?

These scenarios are not finite. AMD affects every aspect of the sufferer's life and a bereavement process is experienced when any kind of visual loss occurs.

Patient support

Access to a counselling facility after unwanted bad news is delivered is essential in order for the patient to begin to reconcile the loss of vision and all that that will mean to them (Barry *et al.*, 2007). Some units will have a service to meet this need but many will not. This is where it may be advantageous for nurses to develop basic counselling skills to enable our patients to begin the grieving journey and to provide information and initiate referral to other 'helping organisations' either charitable or statutory.

Visual impairment and registration

Due to a perceived stigma about being labelled 'disabled', many patients decide not to be placed on the 'sight impaired' or 'severely sight impaired' registers. It is important to emphasise that non-registration is not going to prevent access to agencies that are able to help them. It is essential to explain that it is a government-driven initiative that ensures the availability of funding for service development and provision for all registered patients in their area. Eligibility and access to financial benefit will be blocked through non-registration.

References and further reading

Age-Related Eye Disease Research Group (2001). A randomised, placebo controlled clinical trial of high dose supplements with vitamin C and E, beta-carotene and zinc for age-related macular degeneration and visual loss. *Archives of Ophthalmology*, 119, 1417–36.

Aggawal, R. (2009). *New treatment for dry AMD (IOL Vip)*.
Available at: http://www.66vision.co.uk/#/iol-for-dry-amd/4527060544 (last accessed August 2009).

Antoniak, K., Bienias, W. and Nowak, J. (2008). Age-related macular degeneration – a complex genetic disease. *Klinika Oczna*, 110(6), 211–18).

Baird, P., Robman, L., Richardson, A., *et al.* (2008). Gene-environment interaction in progression of AMD: The CFH gene, smoking and exposure to chronic infection. *Human Molecular Genetics*, 17(9), 1299–1305.

Barry, W., Rovner, B., Casten, R., *et al.* (2007). Dissatisfaction with performance of valued activities predicts depression in age-related macular degeneration. *International Journal of Geriatric Psychiatry*, 22(8), 789–93.

Bressler, S., Munoz, B., Solomon, S. and West, S. (2008). Racial differences in the prevalence of age-related macular degeneration: the Salisbury Eye Evaluation (SEE) Project. *Archives of Ophthalmology*, 126(2), 241–15.

Cong, R., Zhou, B., Sun, Q., Gu, H., Tang, N. and Wang, B. (2008). Smoking and the risk of age-related macular degeneration: a meta-analysis. *Annals of Epidemiology*, 18(8), 647–56.

Da Cruz, L. (2007). *AMD National Knowledge Week, 18–24 June 2007: Surgical intervention: Macular translocation. Eyes and Vision.* Eyes and Vision Specialist Library: National Library for Health.
Available at: http://www.library.nhs.uk/eyes/viewResource.aspx?resID = 261333 (last accessed August 2009).

Evans, J. (2006). Antioxidant vitamin and mineral supplements for slowing the progression of age-related macular degeneration. *The Cochrane Library*. NHS Evidence. Available at:
http://mrw.interscience.wiley.com/cochrane/clsysrev/articles/CD000254/frame.html (last accessed August 2009).

Feskanich, D., Cho, E., Schaumberg, D., Colditz, G. and Hankinson, S. (2008). Menopausal and reproductive factors and risk of age-related macular degeneration. *Archives of Ophthalmology*, 126(4), 519–24.

Friedman, E. (2008). The pathogenesis of age-related macular degeneration. *American Journal of Ophthalmology*, 146(3), 349–89.

Haque, K. (2007). Macular degeneration, symptoms, signs and diagnosis. *Hospital Pharmacist*, 14, 151–53.
Available at: www.pharmj.com/pdf/hp/200705/hp_200705_symptoms.pdf (last accessed August 2009).

Javitt, J., Zhou, Z., Maguire, M., Fine, S. and Willke, R. (2003). Incidence of exudative age-related macular degeneration among elderly Americans. *Ophthalmology*, 110(8), 1534–39.

Johnson, E. (2005). Obesity, lutein metabolism, and age-related macular degeneration: a web of connections. *Nutrition Reviews*, 63(1), 9–15.

Kaiser, P. (2008). Ranibizumab: The evidence of its therapeutic value in neovascular age-related macular degeneration. *Core Evidence*, 2(4), 273–94.

Klein, R., Klein, B. and Linton, K. (1992). Prevalence of age-related maculopathy: the Beaver Dam Eye Study. *Ophthalmology*, 99(6), 933–43.

MacLaren, R. and Pearson, R. (2007). Stem cell therapy and the retina. *Eye*, 21(10), 1352–59.

Mann, S. (2007). Diagnosis – What is OCT. Eyes and Vision Specialist Library. *National Knowledge Week, 18–24 June 2007*. Available at: http://www.library.nhs.uk/eyes/ViewResource.aspx?resID = 261978 (last accessed August 2009).

National Institute of Clinical Excellence (2008). *Implantation of lens systems for advanced age-related macular degeneration*. Available at: http://www.nice.org.uk/Guidance/IPG272/Guidance/pdf/English (last accessed August 2009).

Nursing and Midwifery Council (2008). *Standards of Conduct, Performance and Ethics for Nurses and Midwives*. London: NMC.

Owen, C., Fletcher, A., Donoghue, M. and Rudnika, A. (2003). How big is the burden of visual loss cause by age-related macular degeneration in the United Kingdom? *British Medical Journal*, 87, 312–17.

Rein, D., Saadine, J., Wittenborn, J., *et al.* (2007). Cost effectiveness of vitamin therapy for age-related macular degeneration. *Ophthalmology*, 114(7), 1319–26.

Rutherford, D. (2007). *Antioxidants and oxidative stress*. Available at:
http://www.netdoctor.co.uk/focus/nutrition/facts/oxidative_stress/oxidativestress.htm (last accessed August 2009).

Scott, M., Brown, G., Ho, A., Huang, S. and Recchia, F. (2008). Anti-vascular endothelial growth factor pharmacotherapy for age-related macular degeneration: a report by the American Academy of Ophthalmology. *Ophthalmology*, 115(10), 1837–46.

Tan, J. (2008). Dietary antioxidants and the long-term incidence of age-related macular degeneration: The Blue Mountains Eye Study. *Ophthalmology*, 115(2), 334–41.

Wormald, R., Evans, J., Smeeth, L. and Henshaw, K. (2007). Photodynamic therapy for neovascular age-related macular degeneration. *Cochrane Database of Systematic Reviews*, Issue 3, CD002030, DOI 10.1002/14651858.

Zarbin, M. (2004). Current concepts in the pathogenesis of age-related macular degeneration. *Archives of Ophthalmology*, 122, 598–614.

Abstract available at: http://archopht.ama-assn.org/cgi/content/abstract/122/4/598 (last accessed August 2009).

Useful web resources

66 Vision
http://www.66vision.co.uk/

Bandolier
http://www.medicine.ox.ac.uk/bandolier/
Evidence-based health studies on photodynamic therapy for macular degeneration.

Good Hope Hospital
http://www.goodhope.org.uk/
Macular disease and hints on coping with poor vision.

Macular Degeneration Support
http://www.mdsupport.org/library.html
Search for the article by Roberts on photodynamic therapy.

Macular Disease Society
http://www.maculardisease.org/

National Institute of Clinical Excellence
http://www.nice.org.uk/
Contains an appraisal consultation document on ranibizumab and pegaptanib for age-related macular degeneration, and guidance on implantation of lens systems for advanced age-related macular degeneration.

Net Doctor
http://www.netdoctor.co.uk/

NHS Evidence: Health Information Resources (formerly National Library for Health)
http://www.library.nhs.uk/Default.aspx

RNIB UK Vision Strategy
http://www.rnib.org.uk/xpedio/groups/public/documents/code/InternetHome.hcsp
A fundamental right to sight. A contribution to the National Service Framework for older people and long-term conditions, and independence, well-being and choice.

Royal College of Ophthalmologists
http://www.rcophth.ac.uk/
Visual impairment certification and registration process.

Royal National Institute for the Blind
http://www.rnib.org.uk/xpedio/groups/public/documents/code/InternetHome.hcsp
This has clear information about age-related macular degeneration.

The Eye Digest
http://www.ageingeye.net/
Look for information on Lucentis™ (ranibizumab) for treatment of wet macular degeneration.

United States National Eye Institute
http://www.nei.nih.gov/health/
Facts about age-related macular degeneration.

SELF TEST Answers on page 206

1. Name two possible contributing factors to the development of AMD.

2. Which is the commonest type of AMD – wet or dry?

3. Give two possible symptoms of AMD.

4. What tests could you be asked to do prior to the ophthalmologist's examination of a patient who might have AMD?

5. Which tests might the ophthalmologist require to establish the diagnosis of wet AMD?

6. What health advice might be given to patients with wet AMD?

7. Which drug treatment is currently endorsed by NICE for wet AMD?

8. Following injection treatment for AMD, what adverse symptoms should a patient report urgently?

Chapter 13

Ophthalmic equipment

Sue Cox

Introduction

A wide range of equipment is used in the diagnosis, assessment and monitoring of ophthalmic conditions. It ranges from small optical lenses to large specialist cameras, lasers and field-testing machines. While much of the equipment will be used or operated by the doctor or photographer, some nurses and technicians are trained to operate them too. It is important that you can recognise these items and that you have a basic understanding of what each item is used for and how it is implemented. Such knowledge can allow you to anticipate what may be needed in an examination and will help you to prepare and reassure the patient.

The exophthalmometer

The exophthalmometer is a device used in ophthalmic examination to measure proptosis or exophthalmos, an anterior protrusion of the globe. The most commonly seen cause of proptosis is thyroid eye disease (TED). In this condition, inflammation of the extraocular muscles and orbital fat causes an anterior displacement of the globe within the bony orbit. Other less common causes include orbital tumours and air or blood in the orbit. The degree of ocular protrusion in a normal eye, as measured from the lateral orbital rim to the corneal apex, should read 14–21 mm in an adult. A measurement of greater than 21mm or a difference of more than 2mm between the eyes is generally considered abnormal.

The exophthalmometer is a small hand-held instrument as shown in Fig. 13.1. It consists of a horizontal bar with a yoke

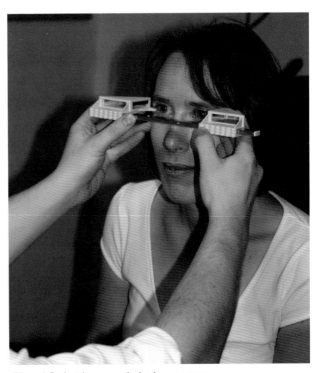

Fig. 13.1 *The exophthalmometer*

mounted at each end, one of which is adjustable to permit movement of the yoke along the bar. Each yoke consists of a notch to allow for alignment with each lateral orbital rim and mirrors for observation of the corneal apex. The horizontal bar is ruled with millimetre gradations for measurement.

The practitioner sits face to face and at eye level with the patient. The instrument should be held with the bar towards the practitioner and with the mirrors at the top. The notches should be placed against the lateral orbital rims. The patient is instructed to look straight ahead. The practitioner then closes the opposite eye to that which is being measured and looks into the mirror on that side. An image of the patient's cornea will be reflected in the mirror. A coloured marker in the mirror housing should be aligned with the corneal apex. The position of this mark can then be measured against the rule on the horizontal bar. This gives a measurement in millimetres of the degree of protrusion of the globe.

In recording measurements of degrees of proptosis it is important that an initial measurement between each orbital rim is recorded. This can then be used as a baseline measurement for future examinations that may be monitoring changes in the degree of the patient's proptosis.

The optokinetic drum

The optokinetic drum is a device used for the stimulation and assessment of optokinetic nystagmus. Nystagmus can be defined as a repetitive, involuntary, to-and-fro oscillation of the eyes. Nystagmus that occurs in response to a moving object through space is normal and acts to preserve clear vision. The ophthalmologist can observe and classify the degree of fixation, the amplitude and frequency of the oscillation and the plane of the nystagmus by using the drum. This can be helpful in assessing the visual acuity of very young infants and also for the detection of patients feigning blindness. Abnormal responses can indicate brainstem damage, congenital nystagmus, cerebellar disease and demyelination. Nystagmus can also present as a reaction to drugs such as phenytoin, lithium, carbamazepine and barbiturates. A bilateral loss of central vision before the age of 2 years, for example with congenital cataract, will also cause nystagmus.

The optokinetic drum is a hand-held instrument consisting of a handle on which is mounted a rotating cylinder. The cylinder is printed with uniform black and white vertical stripes parallel to the axis of rotation. The patient sits in front of the practitioner and is asked to watch the rotating drum. In normal vision an optokinetic nystagmus will be produced. A patient feigning blindness will be unable to suppress this natural reaction.

The pachymeter

Ultrasonic pachymetry uses echo spike techniques to measure the thickness of the cornea. Corneal measurement is essential in refractive corneal surgery and is becoming increasingly used in the assessment of glaucoma patients. As ultrasonic pachymeters have become more generally used it has become apparent that there is a wider variation in central corneal thickness than previously recognised (Iyamu and Memeh, 2007). Normal central corneal thickness is around 0.50–0.54 mm. Furthermore, measurement of intraocular pressure by Goldman applanation is affected by corneal thickness (Iyamu and Memeh, 2007).

The ultrasonic pachymeter is a small hand-held, battery-operated device. It has a detachable probe that can be removed for cleaning. The patient sits while local anaesthetic eye-drops such as oxybuprocaine hydrochloride 0.4% are instilled. The probe is then applied to the cornea. No fixation is required from the patient. The practitioner can use one corneal location to obtain a set of automatically generated average readings across the cornea. Alternatively, single measurements at positions across the cornea may be obtained.

The direct ophthalmoscope and retinoscope

The ophthalmoscope and retinoscope are hand-held instruments that are used for different purposes, but are often found together on the wall mounting. The ophthalmoscope has a flat oval head containing lenses, a mirror and a light beam. There is also a dial for rotating lenses of different strengths. The retinoscope has a rectangular head that houses a light beam and a mirror. This instrument is used in conjunction with trial lenses.

Direct ophthalmoscope

The direct ophthalmoscope is used to examine the fundus or posterior part of the eye. It will, therefore, allow examination of the retina and retinal blood vessels, the choroid, the optic disc and the macula. Direct ophthalmoscopy is widely used by non-specialist practitioners who do not have access to a slit lamp. It can be used to assess the optic disc, which may be swollen in optic neuropathy or cupped in glaucoma. The condition of the retinal blood vessels could indicate retinal artery or vein occlusions. Haemorrhages may be observed, indicating diabetic retinopathy or retinal vein occlusion. Retinal detachment, tears or holes may also be initially diagnosed. However, direct ophthalmoscopy is insufficient for gaining a good view of the peripheral retina and the patient should be referred for indirect ophthalmoscopy if peripheral pathology or damage is suspected.

To use the ophthalmoscope the practitioner sits or stands adjacent to the eye to be examined, preferably examining the right eye with his right eye and hand, and the left eye with his left eye and hand. The lights in the room should be dimmed. All of the settings on the ophthalmoscope should be set to zero. The patient is instructed to focus on a distant object. When the light is first shone into the pupil a red reflex should occur. If this is not seen, then an opacity in the cornea, a dense cataract or a vitreous opacity is indicated and fundal examination will not be possible. Once the red reflex has been seen, the practitioner moves the ophthalmoscope slowly towards the patient and at about 5 cm from the surface of the eye the retina and the optic disc should come into view. These can then be brought into focus by rotating the dial with the index finger until the most suitable lens is found. After examining the posterior pole the patient is asked to look directly into the ophthalmoscope light. The macula and fovea will then automatically come into view.

Retinoscope

The retinoscope is used to obtain an objective measurement of the refractive error of a patient's vision. It can be useful in refracting patients who are unable to participate in a subjective examination that requires judgement and response from the patient. The practitioner shines the light into the patient's eye and observes the reflection off the retina. By moving the light across the pupil the relative movement of the reflection or reflex can be observed. This is then neutralised by manually placing trial lenses in front of the eye until the most appropriate correction is found.

Indirect ophthalmoscopy

Indirect ophthalmoscopy has the advantage of increasing the practitioner's view of the fundus. It provides a clearer view through corneal opacities and cataracts. The periphery of the fundus can be observed and the contrast of lesions such as naevi is improved.

Indirect ophthalmoscopy can be carried out in two ways, by:

- indirect slit lamp biomicroscopy and
- use of an indirect ophthalmoscope.

Indirect slit lamp biomicroscopy

In this method the patient's pupils are dilated using a mydriatic such as tropicamide 1%. The patient sits at the slit lamp and the practitioner commonly uses a +90 or a +78 dioptre lens to examine the fundus. The image is laterally reversed and inverted. The higher the dioptre of the lens, the lower the magnification, but the greater the field of view. However, the higher the dioptre is, the closer the lens needs to be held to the eye. The eye is examined in all positions of gaze.

The indirect ophthalmoscope

An indirect exophthalmometer is shown in Fig. 13.2. This second method provides a good view of the peripheral retina and is commonly used to diagnose or to confirm diagnosis of retinal detachment, holes or tears. It has the advantage of providing a wide field of view. Again, the patient's pupils are well dilated and the patient is then placed in a supine position. The practitioner places on his or her head an ophthalmoscope mounted on a headband (often referred to as an 'indirect'). A 20 + dioptre lens is used for examining the fundus, giving a greater magnification and which can be held at a greater distance from the eye, thus providing a wider field of view. The practitioner must move his or her head and the lens in various directions to examine the different areas of the retina. As the image seen by the practitioner is inverted, the use of the indirect ophthalmoscope is a complex skill to master.

During the examination the practitioner may use a scleral indenter (usually kept with the 'indirect'). This small metal device fits onto the practitioner's finger like a thimble. It has a small T-shaped probe that can be applied to the outside of the upper eyelid at the margin of the tarsal plate. When gentle pressure is exerted visualisation of the peripheral retina is further enhanced.

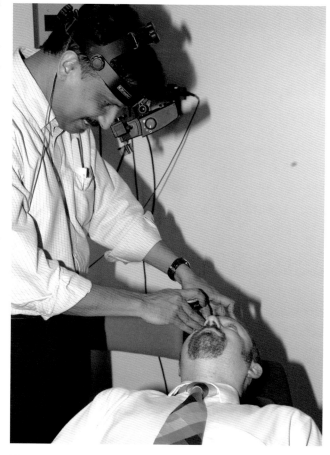

Fig 13.2 *The indirect exophthalmometer.*

The goniolens

Gonioscopy is the examination and analysis of the angle between the posterior corneal surface and the anterior surface of the iris. It provides access to the trabecular meshwork through which aqueous outflow is controlled. Gonioscopy is, therefore, an important element in the examination of patients suspected of having glaucoma.

The most commonly used lens is the indirect gonioscopy lens. The lens has one curved surface, which is applied directly to the cornea like a contact lens. Inside the lens is an arrangement of mirrors which may be a single, double or triple mirror. Mirrors enable the reflection of rays leaving the lens in an approximately perpendicular direction at the contact lens surface. This provides an image in the mirror of the opposite angle.

The patient sits at the slit lamp and a local anaesthetic drop such as oxybuprocaine hydrochloride 0.4% is applied. The practitioner then lubricates the curved surface of the lens with a lubricant like Viscotears™. The patient is asked to look straight ahead and his or her eyelids are held open and the lens tipped so that contact with the cornea is made at the 6 o'clock position, with the mirror at the 12 o'clock position. If a triple-mirror lens is being used, this will be the small domed mirror. The lens is then rotated forward against the cornea and gently pressed against the eye to create a 'suction cup' effect, which keeps it centred on the cornea. Pressure should then be relaxed to avoid distortion of the chamber angle. During examination the lens is rotated clockwise in order that the whole circumference can be viewed.

As well as diagnosis and evaluation of the anterior chamber angle, the goniolens is used in laser procedures. In trabeculoplasty, for example, the use of a triple mirror enables simultaneous visualisation of a wider area of the angle.

The B-scanner

B-scan ultrasonography is a painless and non-invasive method of evaluating the eye in cases where the intraocular structures cannot be visualised. This may be due to corneal opacity, dense cataract or vitreous haemorrhage. It is used for the diagnosis of retinal tears and detachments, particularly where there has been a recent vitreous haemorrhage. It can also be used to detect intraocular tumours and intraocular foreign bodies.

The B-scanner uses ultrasound to produce a two-dimensional display. Ultrasound can be described as an acoustic wave that consists of an oscillation of particles within a medium. Ophthalmic B-scanning focuses a narrow acoustic beam across segments of the retina to produce a two-dimensional sector image. An echo is represented as a dot on the image and the strength of the echo is depicted by the brightness of the dot. The coalescence of multiple dots forms the two-dimensional representation of the examined tissue section.

The patient is asked to sit with his or her eyes closed. Lubricating gel is applied to the scanning sensor, which is then passed over the eyelid. The image produced is shown on a screen and may also be printed out to be kept with the patient's notes.

Fundal photography

The fundus camera is a specialised, low-power biomicroscope with an attached camera that is used for photographing the retina. It is useful for providing a permanent record of the condition of the retina at a point in time, which can then be used for diagnosis and for future comparisons and evaluations.

The camera is mounted on a table that can be pushed towards the seated patient. There is a chin rest and a headband, as on a slit lamp, to help position the patient. Before retinal photography the patient's pupils need to be dilated with a short-acting mydriatic such as tropicamide 1%. The operator sits opposite the patient where the camera's binocular eyepieces and the controls are situated. The camera is connected to a monitor so that the images can be assessed before printing. The optics of the fundus camera work on the principle that the illumination and observation light paths are separate. The observation light, or camera flash, reaches the eye through a series of lenses and a ring-shaped aperture. The reflected light from the retina passes back through the aperture system via two paths, one to the camera and one to the eyepiece.

The fundal camera is used to monitor a number of conditions including glaucoma, diabetic retinopathy, age-related macular degeneration and vascular occlusions. Fundal photography is often used in conjunction with fluorescein angiography as a diagnostic procedure. In this procedure, an intravenous injection of fluorescein 20% (1g per 5 mL) is administered as the patient sits at the camera. As the fluorescein dye flows through the blood vessels of the eye a rapid series of photographs is taken. These record the flow through the choroidal and retinal blood vessels and can indicate areas of vascular leakage, neovascularisation or absence of flow through a vessel.

Adverse reactions to the intravenous injection of fluorescein can occur. Nurses administering the dye should be fully aware of the signs and symptoms of these reactions and be current in their training to deal with them. The nurse should have an 'anaphylaxis box' that contains the appropriate emergency drugs close at hand and they should know the exact whereabouts of the 'crash trolley'. Oxygen and suction should also be readily available.

All patients experience skin discolouration and staining of their urine for about 24 hours following the procedure. A number of patients also experience skin flushing, sometimes accompanied by an itchy rash. They may experience nausea and vomiting. More serious but rarely occurring adverse reactions include laryngeal oedema, bronchospasm and anaphylactic shock.

Angiography may also be performed using a dye called indocyanine green. This is carried out in exactly the same way. This type of angiography is of particular value in studying the choroidal circulation. Adverse side effects are less common with this dye, however it does contain 5% iodine so should not be administered to patients with a known allergy. It is also contraindicated in pregnancy. Common side effects are nausea, vomiting, sneezing and pruritis. Less common are syncope, pyrexia, back ache, skin eruptions and localised skin necrosis.

These symptoms should be outlined to the patient while gaining written consent for the procedure. A detailed history should also be taken, including any known allergies, cardiovascular conditions and details of previous diagnostic procedures using fluorescein or indocyanine green.

Retinal imaging

Specialist imaging devices are used increasingly in ophthalmic examinations and assessments. Two devices in common use are the Heidelberg retina tomograph (HRT) and the optical coherence tomograph (OCT). These also provide a record of the advance of disease, which can inform clinical management.

Heidelberg retina tomograph

This confocal scanning diode laser assesses the optic nerve head by creating a three-dimensional image. It is primarily used for the assessment and management of patients with glaucoma as it can measure the optic disc and the nerve fibre layer. In this system, a laser beam scans the fundus and the amount of light reflected from each scanned point is measured. The fundus is scanned sequentially at depths ranging from 0.5 mm to 4.0 mm, at 0.5 mm increments, producing a layered three-dimensional image. It uses a low light intensity and images can be obtained through an undilated pupil. HRT can only act as part of the examination of the glaucoma patient; clinical assessment of the optic nerve head, field testing and the measurement of intraocular pressure must still be integrated into the diagnosis and monitoring.

Optical coherence tomograph

This is designed to provide high-resolution cross-sectional images of the retina. It operates on the same principle as ultrasound but uses an infrared light beam rather than acoustic waves. The image produced is a map of the intensity of the light reflected from the tissue structures of the retina. Different layers of the retina can be viewed because different tissue structures reflect the light with different intensities. The image produced is not affected by the refractive status of the eye, however the patient's pupils do need to be dilated with a short-acting mydriatic such as tropicamide 1%. The method is useful for diagnosing and monitoring a range of ophthalmic conditions including age-related macular degeneration, central serous retinopathy, choroidal neovascularisation, macular oedema, glaucoma and optic nerve disorders. Even though it is still an emerging technique, it has the potential to reduce the need for more invasive assessments such as fluorescein angiography.

The Humphrey field analyzer

The Humphrey visual field analyzer (Fig. 13.3) is commonly used in the clinical assessment of a patient's visual field. This assessment is termed perimetry. It assesses the degree of any field loss and is most frequently used in the monitoring of glaucoma. Other disease such as retinochoroidal lesions, optic nerve disease and neurological pathology will also produce characteristic patterns of field loss, which can be assessed with perimetry.

The Humphrey field analyzer is an automated perimeter with an in-built computer that enables it to produce detailed and accurate results. The computer stores an age-match set of normal values so that results are presented as a comparison with normal values. It has the ability to automatically re-test abnormal results. The patient's fixation is constantly monitored and poor fixation performance is recorded on the printed result. The Humphrey field analyzer provides an objective assessment because it contains no bias from an examiner.

It is the nurse's or technician's responsibility to supervise the field test and it is important that clear and concise instructions are given to the patient and that their progress is monitored closely. First the patient details, including name, date of birth and hospital identification number are entered into the computer. The patient sits close to the field machine, which is then adjusted to the most comfortable height. The chin rests on an adjustable rest and the forehead is placed against a band, to help maintain the correct position.

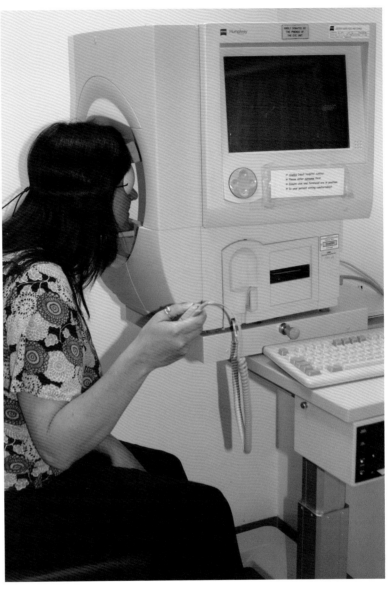

Fig. 13.3 *Humphrey field analyzer.*

One eye is tested at a time, starting with the right. An eye patch is placed over the left. It should be explained to the patient that they need to fix their gaze on the central yellow light, which they will see on the 'field'. Lights of varying intensity will appear across the 'field'. The patient is given a handset and instructed to press a button every time they see one of these lights. They should be reassured that they can blink, and that each point of light is shown more than once. It should be emphasised that their gaze should remain fixed centrally. As the nurse supervises the test, the position of the gaze can be checked on the monitor. Depending on which field test is being carried out, and on the patient's ability and sight, the test for each eye will last for about 4 minutes. When the patient has completed the test the results are saved electronically and printed out to be attached to the patient's notes.

Ideally, the test should be carried out using near-vision correction and there is provision on the analyser for the placement of the appropriate lens in front of the eye. If lenses are not available, the test can be carried out with the patient's own reading spectacles.

To do ...

Visual field defects are not always a result of glaucoma. Make a list of other causes of field loss.

Find out how to check the 'reliability parameters' on the Humphrey visual field test printout.

The patient sits close to and in front of a 'field' on which light stimuli are shown at predefined locations. The stimuli are of increasing or decreasing intensity and the printout plots a 'map' of the patient's visual field. Defects can then be identified. The test determines the severity of field loss in terms of its size, shape and depth. Future tests can then determine the stability or progression of disease.

The predefined pattern of stimuli presented to the patient is termed an algorithm and several different algorithms can be presented by the Humphrey field analyzer. The Central 24-2 test is commonly used for glaucoma monitoring. This test reduces the test time without compromising its ability to detect glaucomatous field loss. The 24-2 test evaluates the temporal 24 degree and the nasal 30 degree areas of the visual field. Other algorithms which you may see used are the 76, the Central 30-2 (which evaluates points up to 30 degrees away from the centre of fixation) and the Estermann binocular field. This field is used to test the patient's field of vision for driving to the standard required by the DVLA and is performed using both eyes simultaneously and with the patient wearing the glasses they have been prescribed for driving.

Recordings of the results are plotted in decibels. They are written as a number between 1 and 40, which represent sensitivity to the stimulus. Sensitivity recorded at around 30 dB is considered to be within normal limits.

Test reliability can be affected adversely by several factors and it is the responsibility of the person supervising the test to minimise them. Improper or erratic fixation can render the test results meaningless, so the patient must be regularly observed on the monitor to check that the examined eye is centrally fixated. Fatigue and anxiety can also affect the result, so it is important that the supervisor explains the test and what is required of the patient clearly and simply. It is useful to select the shortest test appropriate for the patient. Ensure that the patient is sitting comfortably and that the field analyzer is at a suitable height and distance. If vision correction is used it must be ensured that this is correct, either by autorefraction or by lens analysis. When positioning the corrective lens it must be close to the eye, and a lens with a narrow rim suitable for field testing should be used. Broad lens rims and lenses situated too far away from the eye show up on the test results as peripheral field defects. Ptosis or particularly 'heavy' upper eyelids may also show up as field defects or 'artefacts'. Lids can be taped to hold them up during the test.

Regular field testing, performed at least yearly, has become an integral part of the monitoring of glaucoma patients. The visual field defects seen in glaucoma patients have a characteristic appearance and, with clinical examination of the optic disc and the measurement of intraocular pressure, the results can be used to evaluate the efficiency of treatment and the progression of the condition.

Ophthalmic lasers

'Laser' is an acronym for 'Light Amplification by Stimulated Emission of Radiation'. It is essentially a destructive treatment in which ocular pigments absorb light energy and convert it into heat. The laser produces a beam that can deliver a large amount of light energy to a small target area. This causes a therapeutic burn, with minimal damage to the surrounding tissue. There are several laser types in common use in ophthalmology, each used for different treatments. The two most frequently used are the argon laser and the YAG laser.

- The argon laser uses ionised argon as the active medium and produces a beam in the bluegreen visible light spectrum. This is used to perform photocoagulation. It may be used in the treatment of glaucoma, diabetic retinopathy and for retinal holes and tears and repair of detachments.
- The YAG laser uses yttrium-aluminium-garnet as the active medium and produces a beam in the near infrared spectrum. This is used for both photo ablation (the destruction of cells) and photocoagulation. It is used for posterior capsulotomy after cataract surgery and for laser iridotomy for the management of glaucoma.

Other lasers you may see used are the diode laser and the krypton laser. The diode laser uses a semiconductor as the active medium and is used for photocoagulation. Specialist diode lasers can be used to produce low-level non-thermal light to activate the drug Verteporfin (Visudyne™) in photodynamic therapy (PDT) and for transpupillary thermotherapy (TTT) in the treatment of age-related macular degeneration. The krypton laser uses krypton ionised by an electric current as the active medium and produces a beam in the yellowred visible light spectrum. It is used for photocoagulation in retinal disease.

For laser therapy, the patient sits at a slit lamp to which the laser is attached. If the nurse is going to stay with the patient throughout the laser treatment she or he will need to wear special protective glasses. These are green for YAG laser procedures and red for argon laser procedures. For posterior capsulotomy and for retinal photocoagulation treatments the pupils need to be dilated with tropicamide 1%; the doctor may request the addition of phenylephrine 2.5% to ensure good dilation. Topical local anaesthetic drops such as oxybuprocaine hydrochloride 0.4% or tetracaine hydrochloride 1% may also be prescribed.

In posterior capsulotomy, a small opening is created through the opaque growth of epithelial cells across the posterior capsule by a series of short bursts of laser energy. For argon laser trabeculoplasty and iridotomy, performed in the treatment of glaucoma, the pupil must be miosed so the iris is stretched. This reduces its thickness and thus facilitates penetration by the laser beam. Topical pilocarpine 1% or 2% is used in conjunction with a topical local anaesthetic. The doctor may also request topical apraclonidine 1% and oral acetazolamide 250 mg prior to the laser treatment to prevent elevation of the intraocular pressure. A specialised 66-dioptre goniolens with an off-centre planoconvex button is used for iridotomy. For trabeculoplasty, a one- or three-mirror gonioscopy lens is used. The application of a goniolens stabilises the eye, focuses the laser beam and provides magnification. It also acts as a heat sink. Retinal laser photocoagulation is used in the treatment of retinal vascular diseases like diabetic retinopathy, choroidal neovascular membranes, retinal tears and some intraocular tumours.

To do ...

Voke (2001) has written a number of clear and detailed articles on lasers and their use in ophthalmology. Search the internet for 'lasers ophthalmology voke OT magazine' to find more.

References and further reading

Aslam, T. and Azuara-Blanco, A. (2001). Visual field testing in glaucoma with the Humphrey visual field analyzer. *Ophthalmic Nursing*, 4(4), 2326.

Byrne, S.F. and Green, R.L. (1992). *Ultrasound of the Eye and Orbit*. St Louis: Mosby Year Book.

Iyamu, E. and Memeh, M. (2007). The association of central corneal thickness with intra-ocular pressure and refractive error in a Nigerian population. *Online Journal of Health and Allied Sciences*. 6(3).
Abstract available at: http://www.ojhas.org/issue23.htm (last accessed August 2009).

Kanski, J. (2003). *Clinical Ophthalmology*, 5th edn. Oxford: Butterworth Heinemann.

Kwon, Y.H., Fingert, J. and Greenlee, E. (2006). *A Patient's Guide to Glaucoma. Iowa:* University of Iowa. *A simple guide to the visual loss from glaucoma and a guide to the Humphrey automated field test, showing how the POAG field is assessed.*

Lester, M., Garway-Heath, D. and Lemij, H. (eds). (2005). *Optic Nerve Head and Retinal Nerve Fibre Analysis.* Savona: European Glaucoma Society.

Marsden, J. (2007). *An Evidence Base for Ophthalmic Nursing Practice.* Chichester: Wiley.

Olson, J. (2003). *Diabetic Retinopathy Screening Services in Scotland: A Training Handbook.* Aberdeen: University of Aberdeen Available at: http://www.ndrs.scot.nhs.uk/Train/Handbook/drh-00.htm (last accessed August 2009).

Romany, T. and Harvey, B. (2006). Slit lamp biomicroscopy. *Optician*, 232(6069), 2024.

Traverso Carlo, T. (2003). *Terminology and Guidelines for Glaucoma.* 11th edn. Savona: European Glaucoma Society.

Voke, J. (2001). Lasers and their use in ophthalmology, *Optometry*, May 18, 2931

Useful web resources

Eye Casualty
http://www.eyecasualty.co.uk/

Chapter 14

Basic ophthalmic procedures

Dorothy Field

The information in this chapter aims to help guide the beginner in ophthalmology who may want to 'read up' a procedure before they see or learn about it in practice. It is also intended to reinforce what has already been experienced. It is not intended to be prescriptive, as there may be other (possibly better) ways of approaching the areas described that are equally satisfactory. You will of course, always rely on your mentor or another experienced nurse to supervise your practice of each of these procedures until you are assessed as competent to carry them out without supervision. Always ask for help if you are unsure or meet unexpected difficulties.

Make sure you keep your hands in 'good condition' for your job, making regular use of hand creams to prevent cracks and rough areas (most minor ophthalmic interventions are 'clean' rather than completely sterile). Short, well-trimmed nails are important too.

Most of the procedures described in this chapter are carried out in the outpatient department. Rose (2000) comments that due to changes in the NHS these departments are extremely busy and often the numbers of trained ophthalmic nurses have failed to keep pace with demand. Task allocation and the devolution of Snellen testing to capable healthcare assistants (HCAs) means there is little opportunity for a designated nurse or optometrist to follow a patient through their appointment and offer reassurance and explanations about what is happening. In an earlier study, Rose *et al.* (1997) showed how a visual impairment could have profound psychosocial implications. They believed that nurses had an additional responsibility – beyond mere tasks – to help patients adapt to their long-term or short-term visual disability. For these reasons, healthcare assistants should be encouraged to attend 'in house' ophthalmic courses, relevant study days, and to progress with their national vocational qualifications (NVQs) as their informed involvement is essential for excellent patient care, the smooth running of the department, and the identification and transmission of relevant patient issues to the nurse or professionals allied to medicine (PAMs) responsible.

Informed consent is important prior to commencing any ophthalmic procedure, however small it might be. Make sure that you are familiar with the differences between patient compliance, implied consent and informed consent. Good information and the opportunity for the patient to ask questions are critically important. Make sure that the patient makes a clear verbal affirmation of their consent before you begin any intervention.

For the purposes of clarity, the diagnostic tests and procedures that follow below are arranged in the following sections:

1. *Diagnostic tests* (vision tests, tests for possible infection, functional tests (tear production and drainage), measurements of intraocular pressure, the assessment of pupil reactions).

2. *Slit lamp examination.*

3. *Eye care* (cleaning a patient's eyelids, eye-drop and ointment instillation, application of an eye pad, insertion of a bandage contact lens, teaching eyelid taping).

4. *Minor treatments* (eyelid eversion, concretion removal, eyelash epilation, removal of a corneal foreign body).

These are described in varying levels of detail and are meant to be guides rather than complete behavioural descriptions, as they are intended for qualified professional people who are accountable for their clinical practices. It is also recognised that local practices may vary slightly. All these procedures should be taught, supervised and assessed as part of a structured development programme.

1. DIAGNOSTIC TESTS

The following tests are ones that nurses, HCAs and PAMs may be involved in as part of patient 'work up' towards an eventual diagnosis. Tests for basic visual acuity (such as the Snellen, LogMAR or Sheridan–Gardiner) are carried out every time a patient visits an eye department to evaluate whether an ongoing condition has improved, or is stable or has deteriorated. All of these tests look apparently simple to administer, but they require considerable experience in practice to produce accurate results.

The Snellen test

The Snellen chart provides a relatively quick check of central vision, a significant consideration in a busy clinic. It is easy to teach the use of the Snellen chart to new staff, and it is used within hospitals, optometric practices, schools and GP surgeries. It displays standard letters of the alphabet in decreasing sizes. These letters are numbered from 60 at the top, down to 4 or 5 at the bottom, and are printed in black on a white background. The chart needs to be well lit for test purposes, and is designed to be read at a distance of 6 metres. In a small space, this distance can be 'doubled' by the use of an appropriate mirror. It is also possible to obtain 'reduced' charts that can be read at 3 or 4 metres.

How to test vision

Vision testing should be carried out in a private area. The patient should be able to concentrate on the task without any interruptions and without feeling embarrassed that they cannot see well, or do not know the letters, or do not speak English.

Seat the patient 6 metres away from the chart and note if they are wearing contact lenses. Make sure that they put on their bifocals or distance glasses if they have them. If the patient is confused about the terms 'distance glasses' or 'reading glasses' ask them if they have glasses for driving or watching television, and if so, to put them on. Use a disinfected occluder or ask the patient to gently cover one eye at a time, with a cupped hand, and to read out what they can see, beginning at the top of the chart. Make sure that each eye is properly covered throughout the test.

The result for a person with average (or corrected) eyesight is usually around 6/6. In this case, the 6 at the top of the fraction is the number of metres the patient was sitting away from the chart;

the bottom 6 is the size of letters the person with average sight would be able to see from 6 metres away from the chart.

If a very myopic (short-sighted) person was only able to read the large letter at the top of the chart, their vision would be recorded as 6/60. The top figure is still 6 (because the person is still 6 metres away from the chart) but the bottom figure is now 60, indicating that this person is only able to see what the average person (with 6/6 vision) would be able to see from a distance of 60 metres from the chart. (As explained above, each line on the chart is labelled with a tiny number underneath that indicates the distance at which the letters can be read by an average-sighted person.)

Always remember when you are recording a person's right and left visual acuity (RVA and LVA, respectively) to state whether it was with glasses or contact lenses (aided) or without glasses (unaided).

> Record the results as:
>
> RVA 6/12   LVA 6/18 (unaided)
>
> RVA 6/6   LVA 6/9 (with glasses or contact lenses)

Be positive. Someone with healthy eyes may only be able to see for example 6/12 without glasses, but may even manage to see as far as the 6/4 line with glasses or contact lenses. It does not mean that their eyes are 'bad' or 'weak'.

> Children do not like to get tests 'wrong'. If you are using a Snellen chart, it is possible that the letters on the first chart have been memorised by the child, so turn the chart to a fresh set of letters.

Pinhole

Visual acuity at 6/12 or lower is also tested through a pinhole occluder to see whether the person needs spectacles, or whether the low visual acuity results from injury or disease. If a person needs spectacles, use of a pinhole will increase the visual acuity by two lines or so. The pinhole is also useful for testing someone who failed to bring their distance glasses with them. Additionally, if the patient's pupil has been dilated, the lens in the eye may be less able to accommodate, and the vision may be 'down' as a result. Check with a pinhole to see if this makes any improvement. Record your findings.

The following abbreviations will help you record your observations accurately:

Count fingers (CF): When a patient is unable to see the top letter (60) at 6 metres, a hand with outstretched fingers is held in front of him or her and is read, if successful, as Count Fingers (CF at 1 metre, or CF at 0.5 metre).

Hand movements (HM): If the patient cannot manage Count Fingers, check if they can see a hand waving in front of them and record it as HMs. Check in all quadrants of vision, as the patient may also have large visual field defects.

Perception of light (PL): Finally, check if the patient can perceive light in response to flashes from your pen torch in the four quadrants. NPL No Perception of Light

Other abbreviations are:

Pinhole (PH)

Glasses (Glss)

Vision tested without glasses, i.e. unaided (U/A)

Artificial eye (AE)

Record the results as:

RVA *6/6 with glasses*   LVA *CF*
                                     6/60 PH

Lazy (amblyopic) eye

Occasionally you will meet a patient who has one eye that is 'weaker' than the other. They may state that they were treated for 'squint' in childhood. Because at one stage the eye was misaligned, and still might be, the brain never received a clear image on this side, and vision perception did not develop as well as it might have done. There is no treatment for this poor vision in the adult (although a cosmetic re-alignment of the eyes is sometimes carried out).

Always document the 'lazy eye' as

6/12 (patient says lazy eye).

Driving vision

Visual field defects need to be assessed in a hospital ophthalmic outpatient department according to the classes of vehicles specified in the individual's driving licence. This is significant for people with primary open-angle glaucoma. The Driving and Vehicle Licensing Agency (2009) also stipulates the ability to read a standard number plate in good lighting conditions, using both eyes, at 20.5 metres – roughly equivalent to reading 6/10 on a Snellen chart with both eyes. Standard charts do not have a 6/10 line, so test the patient with both eyes uncovered if you are in doubt. Inform the patient if you feel their eyesight may not reach the driving standard, and suggest that they go for a more accurate check with an optometrist once their acute eye condition has settled.

To do ...

Find out what specific area of vision the Snellen chart tests. Are there any disadvantages to the Snellen test?

The LogMAR chart

The ongoing debate

Hussain *et al.* stated: 'The Snellen chart is still widely used within ophthalmology to provide a measure of central visual acuity despite evidence to show its poor reliability and reproducibility' (Hussain *et al.*, 2006). This article appears to make an irresistible case for changing to logMAR visual acuity measurement, but you need to consider that there are many types of this chart available. Among them are the Bailey–Lovie, the EDTRS, the Regan and the Waterloo.

Hazel and Elliott (2002) experimented with these four charts and showed that higher scores could be reached using the Regan chart. This led Hussain *et al.* (2006) to caution that the type of chart used and the scoring method is likely to have a significant effect on the results obtained. To add to the confusion, although many ophthalmologists believe logMAR to be the most accurate measure of visual acuity, particularly for scientific studies, Moutray *et al.* (2008) noted that at least 10 % of the authors in their review of 160 clinical studies appeared to have converted Snellen acuity measurements to a logMAR format – which rather contradicts the premise that logMAR is the most accurate measure, particularly for scientific studies.

The logMAR approach

LogMAR is an algorithm for the logarithm of the minimum angle of resolution (MAR). The distance visual acuity of patients assessed using a LogMAR test is expressed as a logarithmic value. Put another way, the smaller the letters on the chart, and the further away they are, the smaller will be the angle presented to the eye by the letters and therefore the smaller the value of the LogMAR score associated with it.

LogMAR charts 'crowd' the letters together, rather like printed documents, and are thus felt to provide more accurate results (Reid, 2006). The patient is asked to read along the letters, starting with the larger ones at the top of the chart. A score is given for each letter that is read correctly. As with the Snellen test, they are encouraged to guess, and the test is stopped when four mistakes are made in one line.

One of the most popular versions is the ETDRS chart. This was developed for the Early Treatment Diabetic Retinopathy Study in the USA. There are several different ways of scoring this test, however. It is being increasingly used in macular degeneration clinics where it is felt that the acuity score may be useful in detecting subtle changes in vision.

More on the Early Treatment Diabetic Retinopathy Study can be found on the National Eye Institute website.

Scoring the LogMar assessment

The most popular means of scoring logMAR charts in the UK appears to be the one used in the Thomson Software Solutions. Thomson's (2005) article is also available. However, you must use the logMAR chart and scoring method specific to your own department. Learn how to use the equipment competently in practice first, and then read Thomson's article and visit the Thomson website.

The Sheridan–Gardiner test

This is useful for children who can recognise letters by shape but are unable to say what they are. It is also useful for testing a people with learning difficulties and non-English-speaking people. It must always be recorded in the patient's notes that the Sheridan–Gardiner test has been used, because the results may differ slightly from the Snellen test.

A book with one letter displayed on each page is held 6 metres away. The child sits with one eye covered on his or her parent's knee, holding a printed card showing six or eight letters. The child is asked to point to the letter that corresponds with the one being held up. The parent confirms whether the correct letter was chosen. The sizes of the individual letters in the book correspond to the sizes of the letters on a Snellen chart, and are scored similarly. As with Snellen testing, ensure privacy for the patient and minimise distractions for the child.

The near (reading vision) test

In the outpatient department it may also be necessary to test the patient's vision using a near vision chart (reading test type). Each eye should be tested separately. Presbyopic patients will require their reading glasses for an accurate test.

Record the smallest line that can be seen with each eye

RE *N4 (with reading glasses)*   LE *N6*

The near vision test type booklet may also include, for example, pages from a telephone directory or a newspaper. so that the ophthalmologist can detect how functionally impaired the patient might be in daily life or at work.

The Ishihara test for colour blindness

Clinic nurses may be required to carry out this test. Congenital colour blindness is most commonly of the red–green deficiency type. Total colour blindness is extremely rare, and is usually accompanied by poor central vision, photophobia and nystagmus. Acquired colour vision defects may be caused by disease of the optic nerve, retina, brain or even as a result of heavy smoking or alcohol intake.

Using the Ishihara test

The test should be undertaken in a well-lit room, preferably in daylight. One eye at a time should be tested. If reading glasses are used, they should be worn. The test instructions state that it should be carried out fairly briskly, allowing only about 3 seconds to read the number on each plate. There are 25 plates in the Ishihara test-plate book, which should be stored in its cardboard sleeve, out of direct sunlight, as fading may occur.

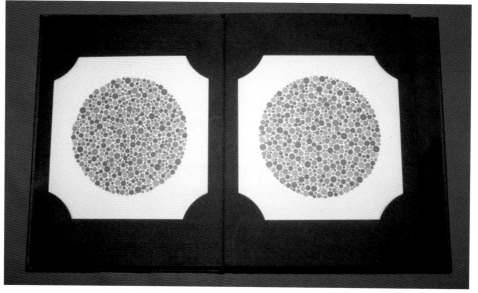

Fig. 14.1 *The Ishihara test (P7)*

The colour plates

Tiny numbers are printed on the front of each plate; if you cannot read them, remove the plate carefully from the black mount, and a larger number is printed on the back. Test the patient on the first 21 plates. If 17 or more plates are read normally, the colour vision is regarded as normal. If 13 or fewer plates are read normally, colour vision is regarded as deficient.

> Record the results as
>
> RE 12/21   LE 18/21

Specific plates serve different functions:

Plate 1: This is used to detect malingerers. Both normally sighted people and those with any sort of colour deficiency can read this.

Plates 2 to 9: The number is seen by the normally sighted, but a different number is seen by those with red–green deficiency. Those with total colour weakness cannot detect the illustrated number at all.

Plates 10 to 17: Normally sighted people can read all of these. Those with red–green deficiency cannot read them at all.

Plates 18 to 21: A number cannot be seen by those with normal vision, but can be read by people with red-green colour deficiency.

Plates 22 to 25: These plates distinguish between different types of red–green colour deficiency (protanopia, protanomalia, deuteranopia and deuteranomalia).

To do ...

What conditions might impair colour vision later in life?

Think about:

- eye conditions
- chemicals and drugs
- substance abuse.

The Amsler grid

This is used to test macular function or to detect and chart a central blind spot (scotoma). There are two Amsler grids in common use in ophthalmology. The original Amsler grid is black with white lines that form a series of horizontal and vertical lines; these lines form 400 small squares, in the centre of which is a white spot. The modified Amsler chart has black lines on a white background. All the Amsler tests are used for testing the central visual field at reading distance. The patient is asked to use one eye at a time, and to fixate on the central spot.

Testing with the modified (white) chart

Ask the patient to put on their reading glasses. Cover one eye at a time and ask the patient to look at the Amsler grid from a comfortable reading distance. Report on the following:

- Can the patient see the central spot?

- Does the patient perceive the chart as black and white?

- Can they see the four corners of the grid, and the four sides of the grid?

- Do the lines in the grid all look square or are some distorted? Are there any blurred or missing areas? Ask the patient to use your pen or pencil to draw round these areas.

- Do any of the lines appear to be moving? Ask the patient to indicate them.

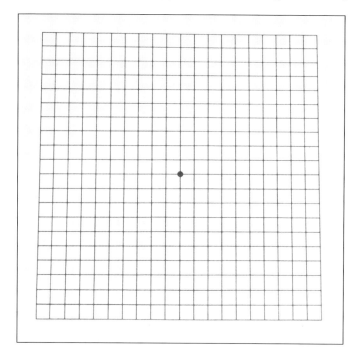

Remember to remind the patient to keep looking at the central dot throughout the test.

The way in which the patient perceives the squares to be altered (a curved perception in a serous retinal separation; a blind spot or scotoma in optic nerve disease) may provide clues towards the patient's provisional diagnosis.

Label the Amsler grids for the left and right eyes, and put the patient's address label on them both. The ophthalmologist will use them in conjunction with ophthalmoscopic examination. Write your findings on the chart or in the patient's notes.

Fig. 14.2 *The modified Amsler grid.*

The Amsler grid may be given to patients with age-related macular disease to take home for self-monitoring. However, the grids are known to be quite unreliable for predicting these retinal changes. In the absence of a better tool, Crossland and Rubin (2007) recommend continued use of it – with the caveat that absence of change detected on the Amsler grid cannot be interpreted as absence of macular degenerative changes.

Tests for possible infections (conjunctival swabs)

Conjunctival swabs for culture

You will need:

- the patient's notes

- the correct laboratory request forms

- the correct culture media (e.g. charcoal media, viral transport media, Chlamydia media)

- sterile dry swabs

- box of paper tissues

- a minim of saline

- a minim of hydroxymethylcellulose

- a minim of oxybuprocaine hydrochloride 0.4 %.

Basic ophthalmic procedures

It is a good plan to complete the correct laboratory request forms and label the containers for the swabs before you fetch the patient, so that you can give the patient your full attention during the procedure. Each label must state:

- the patient's name and date of birth
- whether it is the right or left eye
- the date and time
- the patient's hospital number
- the ward or department name or number (and sometimes the first line of the address)
- the consultant's name.

General principles

Explain to the patient what you are going to do, and seat them comfortably with their head supported. Most ophthalmic nurses use preservative-free oxybuprocaine hydrochloride 0.4% eye-drops as a local anaesthetic prior to this procedure if the patient's eye is very sore. Wolfel *et al.* (2006) and Macdonald and Ramasethu (2007) support this approach. You can moisten the end of the sterile specimen swab you are going to use with a drop from the minim of normal saline (this makes the procedure more comfortable for the patient and will not alter the results, (Cagle and Abshire, 1981; Nayak and Satpathy, 2000).

Never instil fluorescein prior to taking swabs for culture, as *Chlamydia* swabs use cells to culture *Chlamydia trachomatis* by fluorescein antibody staining. It is therefore imperative that this dye is not instilled prior to taking this swab because you could contaminate a complete laboratory test batch.

Bacterial conjunctival swabs

Bacteria are the most common cause of conjunctivitis. Gently pull the lower eyelid down. Ask the patient to look up, and rub the specimen swab inside the lower eyelid from the inner to the outer canthus, using a firm, rotating movement to collect any discharge present (do not touch the eyelid margins). Put the swab into the culture media supplied by your NHS trust. If required, repeat the procedure for the other eye.

Viral conjunctival swabs

Viral swabs must gather as many intact conjunctival cells as possible. Wolfel *et al.* (2006) found that using one drop of preservative-free oxybuprocaine 0.4% prior to sampling resulted in significantly greater numbers of conjunctival cells being obtained from a group of patients with locally anaesthetised eyes than with the matched control group. They state that all the swabs obtained from their test groups were vigorously rubbed over both the upper and lower conjunctival surfaces.

Chlamydia conjunctival swabs

As the area being swabbed for *Chlamydia* needs to be free from mucous and pus, it is wise to always take the bacteriology swab first to prepare the area for this test. It is definitely better to use oxybuprocaine hydrochloride 0.4% eye-drops as a local anaesthetic prior to this test (Macdonald and Ramasethu, 2007) which can be quite painful. Use firm pressure and rotate the moistened swab to obtain a good sample of conjunctival epithelial cells from the bulbar and palpaebral conjunctiva of the upper and lower fornices of the eye.

Following the collection of conjunctival swabs, it is good practice to instil drops of hydroxy-methylcellulose into each eye for comfort (unless the patient is allergic to it). Double check your documentation and labelling prior to bagging the swabs and sending them to the appropriate department. Document in the patient's notes the date, time and type of swabs taken and sign the entry.

Functional tests (production and drainage of tears)

Lacrimal sac syringing and washout

The reasons for carrying out this procedure are generally:

- to check the patency of the tear ducts
- to flush out a small mucoid obstruction (to relieve a watery eye, or epiphora).

Occasionally it is used:

- to introduce dye for a radiographic procedure (e.g. dacryocystogram)
- to flush out purulent matter in chronic dacryocystitis (very dilute antibiotics may be used as part of this process).

You will need:

- a sterile pack containing a paper towel, small swabs and a gallipot opened on a clean surface
- local anaesthetic eye-drops
- a 2 mL syringe
- 5–10 mL sterile saline 0.9% poured into the gallipot
- a disposable lacrimal cannula
- good lighting
- the patient's notes
- an anglepoise lamp.

You may also need:

- a binocular headband loupe
- a Nettleship's dilator (used in some eye units)
- a Hayes punctum seeker
- cotton-wool buds.

Procedure

Position your patient comfortably (on either a couch or semi-reclining in a treatment chair) and explain that you are going to flush out the little drainage pipes in the corners of their eyelids using a small, blunt tube. If the tubes are working, a tiny bit of salty water will be tasted at the back of their mouth, which they should swallow. Make sure that the light is shining into the inner corner (medial canthus) of the correct eye, and with cleaned hands gently pull down the corner of each lower lid to check the size of the lower puncti. If they are difficult to see and possibly stenosed you may require the Nettleship's dilator or the Hayes punctum seeker.

Wash your hands. Instil local anaesthetic drops. Arrange the contents of your sterile pack (preferably out of the patient's line of vision) and draw just over 1 mL saline into your syringe. Attach the lacrimal cannula, and gently press the syringe plunger to ensure that a small stream of saline will readily squirt into the gallipot.

Tuck the paper towel around the patient's neck in case there are any drips. Ask him or her to look up to ensure that the cornea is out of the way, and pull the bottom eyelid down slightly with your thumb to 'anchor' it. Gently introduce the cannula into the lower canaliculus until you feel a 'hard stop'. This is the medial wall of the sac, which lies along the lacrimal bone. Withdraw the cannula slightly so that it is positioned within the lacrimal sac. Squeeze the plunger of the syringe very gently. Normally the solution should dribble into the nasopharynx, at which point the patient reports a salty taste at the back of the mouth or you observe them swallowing. Withdraw the cannula.

> Record this in the patient's notes as:
>
> *Lacrimal duct freely patent.*

Unfortunately this procedure is not always simple. When you are learning and observing it, you will note that the openings to the ducts are often stenosed. Sometimes the lower canaliculus is blocked and you will experience a 'soft stop' to your cannula and see the saline being regurgitated through the lower punctum. If the common canaliculus is blocked, fluid will regurgitate through the upper punctum. When this happens, as the second nurse present you may be asked to press a moistened cotton bud over the upper punctum to occlude it while your more experienced colleague applies gentle force in an attempt to relieve a slight obstruction.

To do ...

Carefully observe and ask questions. Remember how the details of what happened are recorded in the patient's notes.

The Schirmer test

This test is a means of measuring the amount of aqueous tear fluid produced in a given time. It is one of a number of tests that can be used to diagnose the type of 'dry eye' that a person might be suffering from, and is particularly useful for patients with suspected Sjogren's disease.

You will need:

- a box of sterile Schirmer strips
- local anaesthetic eye-drops (if required)
- a kitchen timer.

Procedure

Seat your patient comfortably and explain that you are going to measure the tears they produce using sterile blotting paper. Clean your hands.

You will need to have found out which doctors prefer to have local anaesthetic eye-drops instilled prior to this procedure and remember to use them accordingly. Nurse practitioners seeing their own patients may choose to have this test done, and will need to decide for themselves whether or not to use local anaesthetic drops before testing. Always leave a few minutes between instilling the drops and inserting the Schirmer strips.

> **Reflex** tears (in response to the local irritation of the Schirmer strips) and **basal** tears ('normal' residual tears) are measured when the test is carried out without local anaesthetic.

If you are using local anaesthetic, give the patient a clean tissue and ask them to gently blot their closed eyes once the stinging from the eye-drops has worn off, then place the strips. Ideally, basal tears are measured when local anaesthetic is instilled, but there is still likelihood that some reflex tears will be stimulated.

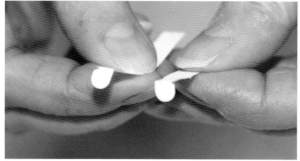

Fig. 14.3 *Folded Schirmer's papers.*

Make sure that your hands are very dry before removing the strips from their sterile packets. Fold each strip over at the notch (Fig. 14.3). You will need to fold them so that the notches will face to the outer canthus of each eye.

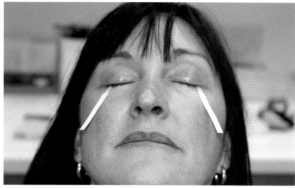

Fig. 14.4 *Patient with Schirmer's papers inserted.*

When your patient is ready, gently insert the papers inside the lower eyelid of each eye, about three-quarters of the distance from the inner canthus (Fig. 14.4).

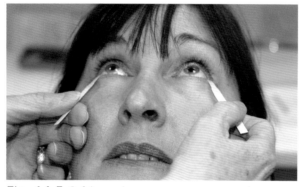

Fig. 14.5 *Schirmer's papers are removed simultaneously.*

Some eye units tell their patients to keep their eyes open, and others require them to be closed. Check local custom before you begin the test. Then, after exactly 5 minutes, carefully remove both papers simultaneously (Fig. 14.5).

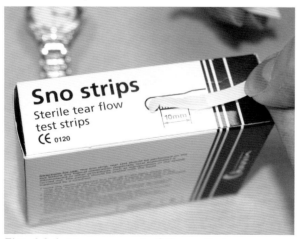

Fig. 14.6 *Measurement of the wetted area of a Sno-strip* (Laboratoire Chauvin, France).

Use the printed measure on the side of the Schirmer strip box to carefully measure the wet area (Fig. 14.6). Record the measurement for the right and left eyes in the patient's notes. A result of less than 5 mm of wetting indicates a dry eye, and about 10 mm is considered normal. Record within the patient's notes the measurements for each eye, how long the strips were in place for, and whether or not local anaesthetic was used. Some ophthalmologists also like to have the strips stuck on to the patient's notes, but mark the wet area with a ballpoint pen first.

The Eye Digest gives more information regarding dry eyes and the tests used to diagnose this condition. It should be noted that some patients with 'dry eyes' actually present with sore, watery eyes and may still produce a good quantity of tears. A tear break-up time (BUT) test with a slit lamp may indicate that the eyes are 'dry' because the other components of the tear film – the mucin layer or the oily film – are not present in sufficient quantities to hold the tear film efficiently on the front of the eye.

Measuring intraocular pressure

The text below describes just some of the methods for measuring intraocular pressure. Learning to measure and accurately record it takes time, patience and good clinical supervision, and the best learning opportunities often arise in glaucoma clinics. These patients are generally familiar with the procedures and are practised at keeping their eyes still and wide open. They are also more likely to allow learners to practise and are often extremely helpful and encouraging towards them.

Goldman applanation tonometry

This measures intraocular pressure. In eye departments, the Goldman tonometer is probably the most frequently used form of applanation tonometry. Applanation relates to the force required to make a reading of the intraocular pressure. Applanation tonometry of the cornea is based on the Imbert–Fick Law (sometimes spelt Imbert–Flick in ophthalmic journal articles) and uses the following formula to produce a reading:

P = F/A

Where P is the pressure within the eye, F is the applanation force and A is the area of constant corneal flattening (3.06mm diameter of area of cornea depressed).

If the patient needs to have their pupil dilated, this test should be carried out first, because in a patient with narrow drainage angles (see Chapter 9) pupil dilatation could result in a higher reading. This procedure should not be carried out if the patient has keratitis or a corneal abrasion, or if you suspect they may have an eye infection.

Intraocular pressure is defined by Witchell (1989) as the pressure within the eye that is influenced by the vitreous humour, which normally remains constant, and the aqueous humour, which is produced by the ciliary body and leaves through the filtration angle and the uveoscleral drainage route. Thus the pressure within the eye results from the balance between aqueous production and drainage.

You will need:

- a slit lamp
- a Goldman applanation tonometer
- a tonometer prism (disposable or cleaned and stored according to local guidelines)
- minims of local anaesthetic (e.g. oxybuprocaine hydrochloride 0.4%) and Fluorets™ or a proprietary mixture of local anaesthetic and fluorescein
- paper tissues.

It is difficult to learn how to achieve accurate pressure readings quickly. You will first need plenty of practice in using a slit lamp to examine the eye in order to develop the fine handling skills and confidence required to obtain a satisfactory reading. Your practice must be supervised until you are consistently accurate. Set yourself up with a notebook, and write the patient's name, date and your readings for each eye. Your supervisor should write their readings beside yours, and sign their entry. It is wise to ensure that your practice is formally certificated in some way before you take measurements without supervision. This will ensure patients receive a high standard of care, and you will have some protection against complaints within the Nursing and Midwifery Council Code 2008 (page 5, para. 2). Keep your skills and knowledge up to date.

Procedure

Clean the slit lamp prior to use. Seat your patient comfortably, at an appropriate height at the slit lamp. Explain what you are going to do. Wash your hands and instil local anaesthetic drops and fluorescein.

Place the tonometer head into the holder (without touching the area that will come into contact with the patient's cornea) with the 0 or 180 lined up with the marks at the top of the holder.

Fit the tonometer on to the slot on the bed of the slit lamp. The right slot is used for the right eye view through the right eyepiece and vice versa for the left eye. Adjust the dial on the side of the tonometer until it reads 10.

Ask your patient to place their chin on the slit lamp rest and their forehead against the bar at the top of the head frame. Switch the slit lamp light on to blue filter, full beam with the slit wide open. Slide the movable base of the slit lamp forward until the tonometer head is close to the eye.

Talk to the patient, reminding them to keep both eyes open, head pressed hard against the headband and to look straight ahead, pretending they are slightly surprised, so that their eyes will be wide open. Using the 'joystick' and under direct vision, edge the tonometer head in to the centre of the cornea. Look through the eyepiece, and place the tonometer on the centre of the cornea (Fig. 14.7).

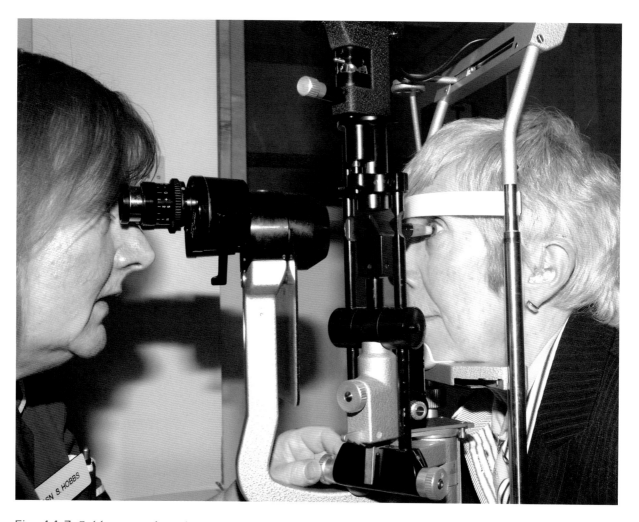

Fig. 14.7 *Goldman applanation tonometry.*

Two half circles should appear in the viewer. Adjust the dial on the tonometer until one half circle is immediately inside the other, just touching, and looks like a prone letter S. Check the reading on the tonometer dial, ask the patient to sit back in the chair and record the reading in the notes. Remove the tonometer head, and either dispose of it or clean and process it as per your local protocol.

 A fully illustrated instruction manual can be downloaded as a PDF from the National Glaucoma Society. Unfortunately this document is in three languages and is lengthy, so it would be better to check first if you have a printed English manual in your department.

Note: It is not advisable to perform applanation on patients with eye infections, corneal abrasions or obvious penetrating injuries.

To do ...

Find out about diurnal variations in intraocular pressure. What factors might cause the intraocular pressure reading to be inaccurate?

Can a nurse inadvertently cause a patient harm while measuring intraocular pressure?

Calibration of Goldman applanation tonometers

A study by Tattersall (2006) attempted to discover whether a protocol for calibration of Goldman applanation tonometers could improve the accuracy of intraocular pressure measurements. It revealed in one large teaching hospital that 62.5% of tonometers had an error of greater than or equal to 1 mmHg. Sandhu *et al.* (2005) recommended that calibration checks should be carried out monthly and any with calibration checks of greater than +/– 2.5 mmHg should be returned to their manufacturers for re-calibration. Immediate checks should be made if tonometers suffer specific damage. In their view, ophthalmologists should ideally check calibration before each session. In some units, tonometers are checked regularly by the departmental optometrist and annually by the manufacturer. A 6-monthly check by the manufacturer had been reduced to an annual check as a 'cost saving' and thus the imperative for regular checks 'in house'.

 The manufacturer's information manual for tonometer calibration can be downloaded from the website of the National Glaucoma Society (USA), but this is not something you should be attempting without education, supervised practice and accreditation of your competence within your ophthalmic unit.

Cleaning applanation tonometer prisms

Hillier and Kumar (2008) in a survey of eye units with training recognition showed that 77% continue to re-use tonometer prisms. Nurses must be aware that there is a theoretical risk of transmitting variant CJD (Creutzfeldt–Jacob disease) from tonometer prisms that are not adequately cleaned. Lim *et al.* (2003) demonstrated that patients using eye-drops regularly desquamated more corneal cells with Goldman tonometry than those not using eye-drops regularly. They found that wiping and washing the tonometer prism immediately after use, before epithelial cells dried on the surface, reduced the cell numbers, but did not eliminate them all; therefore they concluded that retained cells on tonometer prisms might represent potential prion activity. Make sure that you adhere to your local guidelines when cleaning tonometer heads. At the end of the clinic session the prism should be soaked in sodium hypochlorite for at least 5 minutes, rinsed in sterile saline and then stored dry (Hawksworth, 2008).

Disposable tonometer prisms

These have not been without problems. The introduction of disposable prisms has prompted research on their utility. Maino *et al.* (2006a) believed that caution should be exercised when using disposable prisms for pressures in excess of 25 mmHg, but acknowledged their increasing accuracy. A different study by Maino *et al.* (2006b) compared disposable devices, and found the disposable prisms to be much more accurate than silicone shields for non-disposable prisms. Very worryingly, Rajak *et al.* (2006) surveyed staff who used disposable tonometer prisms, and found that 50% of them admitted touching the applanation face prior to using it. Culture of these prisms demonstrated the presence of a range of pathogens.

Personal research suggests that disposable tonometer prisms can be difficult to fit to the tonometer, which may have led to the findings of Rajak *et al.* (2006). However, with a little practice it is possible to fit them without contaminating them.

Disposable prisms are very expensive purchases for an eye unit, and the research by Rajak *et al.* (2006) suggested that unless they are fitted carefully an eye unit might still be at risk of sustaining an adenovirus outbreak, although they pointed out that patients would be protected from the theoretical risk of contracting vCJD. Unless conscientious hand-washing and aseptic techniques are used, this large investment in improving patient safety could be seriously undermined.

Other tonometric measures of intraocular pressure

The TonoPen™

A TonoPen™ is a very small, hand-held instrument, useful for obtaining intraocular pressure readings when a slit lamp is not immediately available. It is good for measuring the intraocular pressure of eyes with corneal irregularities. Readings may be a little higher than those obtained with the Goldman tonometer.

The Perkins tonometer

The Perkins tonometer is a light, hand-held tonometer that operates much like the Goldman tonometer, although more operator expertise is required to achieve an accurate reading. It is suitable for patients who are unable to sit at the slit lamp.

The Schiotz tonometer

The Schiotz tonometer is a very basic instrument for measuring intraocular pressure. It is now mainly used in developing countries because the equipment is relatively cheap and does not require electricity or batteries.

Pneumotonometry

Pneumotonometry is a non-contact method of measuring the pressure of the eye. It does not require the use of eye-drops. A light is shone into the patient's eye, and a puff of air is blown forcefully against the

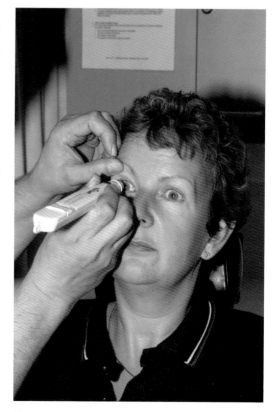

Fig. 14.8 *The TonoPen™*

cornea. The results of this method of measurement are less accurate and less consistent, but they provide useful screening information, particularly for high-street opticians.

Assessing pupil reactions

Relative afferent pupillary defect (RAPD; Marcus Gunn pupil)

This is a test for optic nerve disease. In normal lighting conditions, the patient's pupils appear normal. When a bright light is shone on to them, both pupils will contract. This is called a consensual pupil response.

To carry out this test, arrange very dim lighting conditions and stand slightly to the side of the patient, so that they are not tempted to focus on you, but make sure that you have a good view of the pupils of both eyes. Ask the patient to 'relax' their eyes and pretend that they are looking across to the far side of a field. (You must ensure that the patient has 'relaxed' their focus, because as well as reacting to light, the pupils will also miose when their gaze is fixed on a near object.) When you are sure that the patient is ready, swing a strong light beam into the asymptomatic eye for a second or two. You will see the pupil constrict. Without moving the light beam, observe the affected eye. Because the neural pathways for the asymptomatic eye are functioning, the brain will pick up this impulse and will send a signal to the affected eye, warning it to contract. You can see this happen.

Swing the torchlight slowly on to the affected eye, by dipping the beam below the patient's nose, and then shining it into the affected eye. If the eye problem is with the neural pathway, the damaged pathway will transmit the signal less efficiently and the brain will sense less light entering the eye, so causing both pupils to dilate slightly to let in more light.

Remember that the resting pupil diameter is smaller in elderly people and the response in terms of maximum dilation is smaller (Bitsios et al., 1996), so elderly people are particularly difficult to examine. It is important to check for any RAPD prior to dilating a new patient's pupils for examination. Document that you have done this. If there is a gross problem, this is easy to identify, but sometimes the difference between the reactions in the two eyes is very subtle as mentioned above. You should double check any findings with a more experienced colleague until you are fully competent. If you find an RAPD, speak to the ophthalmologist; he or she may wish to verify your finding of RAPD prior to the pupil being dilated, as this is potentially very significant to the diagnosis, particularly in optic nerve disease.

Pupils equal and reacting to light and accommodation (PERLA)

When you have checked that both pupils are equal, round and reacting to light, you must check the accommodation reflex. Put the room lights on. Sit directly in front of the patient so that you can observe the pupils of both eyes. Hold out your pen (or your finger) in front of both your noses, about 10 cm from the patient's nose. Ask the patient to look at the pen for a few seconds, then into the distance, and then back at your pen. You should be able to see both eyes converging slightly for near vision, straightening up for distance, and converging again for near. Observe the pupils of both eyes simultaneously, and you should see the pupils of both eyes miose slightly, and equally for near vision. This is called the accommodative reflex. If everything is working correctly, you can write down 'PERLA' on the patient's notes.

Recording your findings

If everything is working correctly, you can write down 'PERLA' on the patient's notes. If there is an RAPD, this is recorded as "RAPD' (specify whether the right or left eye is affected).

---

2. SLIT LAMP EYE EXAMINATION

New nurses are often allowed little time by their managers (who may not be ophthalmic nurses) to learn this complex skill. If you are being harassed about being a slow learner, it would be well to remember the following:

- Not all the slit lamps in the department were made by the same manufacturer or have exactly the same controls; they are similar, but you have to learn to use the different types.
- In order to use a slit lamp in the nursing management of a patient's condition, you need to learn the anatomy and physiology of the eye thoroughly and learn about a wide range of conditions first.
- When you start looking through the slit lamp, you must learn to distinguish between the normal and the abnormal. Textbooks have good, clear, carefully chosen pictures of eye problems, but what you see in practice is often more subtle.
- In order to practice effectively – and safely – learning from a well-structured eye course that includes supervised clinical practice and practice assessments is particularly helpful for acquiring slit-lamp skills.

Learning to use a slit lamp depends on practice, like learning to drive a car. Initially you will need to work with an experienced practitioner, but as you progress you will need less supervision (but continue to have your clinical findings checked for patient safety and to learn from what you are seeing). When you reach the final step of working alone, remember that it takes a while to adjust to the responsibility of managing an ophthalmic client group in a nurse-led clinic. Any eye clinic encounters with outpatients (not emergency patients) should begin with the whole patient and gradually focus on the eye. Your welcome to patients should include an assessment of their mood and general health, with open questions that allow them to share information about their general health and their eyes in particular. Check their visual acuity for any changes and their face for any swelling or bruising. Check that both their eyes look 'normal'.

General slit lamp examination

- Check the eyelids for small swellings, blepharitis or discharge. Check that the eyelashes are growing normally. Are the eyelids correctly aligned, or turning in, or drooping away from the eye?
- Check the conjunctiva for haemorrhage or dilated blood vessels (note the location of any hyperaemia). If there is a drainage bleb, you must check that this is adequately formed.
- Check the cornea for a bright corneal light reflex and any obvious opacities. Post surgically you must note if the anterior chamber is formed, and any wound is secure. Stain with fluorescein if necessary. Check the operation site (corneal or scleral) and that the section is intact.
- Check the pupils to see if they are equal and reacting normally. Is there a 'red reflex'? Note the pupil response to any prescribed mydriatics or miotics the patient is taking. Is the pupil an odd shape?
- Check the anterior chamber for hypopyon (pus in the anterior chamber) or hyphaema (blood in the anterior chamber). Check for inflammatory cells in the aqueous by looking in the oblique slit lamp beam under maximum intensity and magnification. The beam should be 1mm wide, and the cells are seen as tiny particles moving slowly through the tiny beam of light. Kanski (2007) suggests that the cells seen in the slit lamp beam should be counted and graded as in Table 14.1.

Table 14.1 *Inflammatory cells seen in the slit lamp beam*

Grade	Cells in field
0	< 1
0.5 +	1–5
1 +	6–15
2 +	16–25
3 +	26–50
4 +	> 50

Aqueous flare is an inflammatory haze in the aqueous. Kanski (2007) similarly advises grading of aqueous flare as shown in Table 14.2.

Table 14.2 *Grading of aqueous flare seen in the slit lamp beam*

Grade	Description
0	Nil
1 +	Faint
2 +	Moderate (iris and lens details clear)
3 +	Marked (iris and lens details hazy)
4 +	Intense (fibrinous exudates)

If you have a local protocol which differs from that above, follow it. Document your examination findings and actions carefully. Always seek a second opinion/advice where necessary.

The Seidel test

This test is carried out at the slit lamp as a diagnostic test. It is used to check for a leaking perforation of the eyeball – either following surgery or following injury. You will need a minim of fluorescein 2%.

Position the patient comfortably at the slit lamp by adjusting the patient chair, the height of the slit lamp and the chin rest. Explain that you are going to instil some yellow eye-drops and that some of the dye may run down the patient's face. Use the blue filter light at maximum light intensity. Obtain a good view of the area you are going to examine by asking the patient to look up, down, to the right, and so on, and to hold the position while keeping their head firmly in the slit lamp head frame. Hold their eyelids open, and drop the fluorescein generously slightly above the area for examination. If fluid is leaking from the eye, it can be seen as a green stream, diluting the fluorescein dye.

A negative Seidel's test is not absolute proof that there is no leak. Record your findings and refer as necessary. This test should only be carried out by learners under the supervision of competent, experienced personnel.

To do ...

As this has been a very brief introduction to the use of the slit lamp, ask an experienced colleague to show you the different ways of adjusting the mirrors, magnification and lights.

Find out the names of the hand held lenses which are used at the slit lamp.

Find out where the spare bulbs are kept, and learn how to change these.

Keep observing the slit lamp in use to find out more about the range of adjustments, and continue asking questions.

3. EYE CARE

Showing patients how to care for their eyes effectively or showing carers how to do this for those who are unable to manage for themselves is most important. Given that many medical interventions are now provided as 'day care', it is essential that good, clear explanations are given to patients or their relatives regarding ongoing eye care, including the reasons as to why the specific care is necessary. The instructions given below are for guidance, but it is accepted that local practice may vary.

Cleaning a patient's eyelids

It is exceptionally uncomfortable to have sticky eyes. The vision blurs periodically, hardened crusts are potential reservoirs of infection, and the hardened exudates can feel very scratchy around the eye. Patients who are able to do so should be encouraged to manage their own eyelid cleansing, but children and their parents may need help and encouragement. Poorly patients need to have this done for them.

You will need:

- a clean working surface
- a sterile gallipot
- sterile saline
- sterile gauze swabs or cotton-wool balls (generally gauze swabs are favoured for eye cleaning post surgery because of the fibrous nature of cotton-wool).

Explain to your patient what you are going to do. If possible, position them so that their head is supported. Wash your hands. Put a little saline into the gallipot and open the packet of swabs. Clean your hands again. Use one finger to pull the patient's lower eyelid down slightly and press against the cheekbone to keep the eyelid still. Ask the patient to look up and gently wipe from the inner canthus to the outer canthus. When you have cleaned the lower lid satisfactorily, begin the top eyelid. This time ask the patient to look down and pull the upper eyelid up gently, securing it with gentle pressure on the upper orbital margin. Wipe gently from the inner to outer canthus as before.

If the eyelids are very stuck together, it is a good idea to leave the patient relaxing comfortably with both eyes closed and a 'sloppy wet' swab over the stuck eyelids for 10 minutes (while you do something else) before you have another gentle try at opening the lids.

To do ...

This task probably represents a lifetime's ophthalmic experience. Not all 'sticky eyes' are infected. The conjunctiva seems to produce a wide range of qualities of secretion depending on the challenges it is facing (e.g. bacterial conjunctivitis, retinal detachment surgery with plomb, viral conjunctivitis, squint surgery). Learn to recognise the 'stickiness' that accompanies each different category of eye problem, so that you can recognise the 'normal' types of stickiness.

Eye-drop and ointment instillation

Eye-drop prescriptions to the uninitiated can be confusing as they are often written thus in ophthalmic settings:

G. chloramphenicol

Gutt. chloramphenicol

Guttae chloramphenicol.

This relates to the tradition of writing prescriptions in Latin. *Gutta* is the Latin word for teardrop, and is used as above to indicate medicines that are administered as eye-drops. Similarly the Latin word *oculentumi* is shortened to *oc.* and *occ.* and is often used in prescriptions for ophthalmic ointment.

Ophthalmic abbreviations in prescriptions

These are a further cause for concern for new staff. Examples are chloramphenicol (Chlor.), homatropine (HA) and phenylephrine (PE). Do find out if your area of practice has an agreed list of abbreviations, and always check when you are unsure. Remember that eye-drops can be as potent as oral medications, because the mucosa of the eyelids, nose and mouth is thin and well vascularised and able to absorb drugs directly into the bloodstream (e.g. like glyceryl trinitrate spray is absorbed directly from the mouth). This route produces a greater pharmacological effect than when drugs are taken orally because the metabolic processes of the intestine and liver do not mediate their effects. Take enormous care particularly with phenylephrine administration in children and the elderly.

Key standards for eye-drop and ointment instillation

Check that the prescription is:

- dated for the patient's current treatment episode
- signed by a doctor, nurse prescriber or a competent nurse acting under a valid protocol.

Also ensure that:

- the dosage is clear
- the correct eye is indicated
- the correct drug is used in the correct concentration for the correct patient.

Make sure the patient has no known sensitivity to the prescribed eye-drop or ointment or to any of its components (e.g. preservatives in eye-drops and the carrier grease in the ointment).

Wash your hands or clean them with antiseptic gel. Hold a clean tissue in one hand and the eye-drops or ointment in the other. Explain to the patient what you are going to do and why. Check whether the eyelashes are crusted and clean them if necessary. Ask the patient to look up so that you do not accidentally abrade the cornea with the eye-dropper or ointment nozzle. Using the tissue to cover the thumb of one hand, gently pull the lower eyelid down and instil one drop into the lower fornix or squeeze about 1 cm of ointment into the lower fornix. The tissue will absorb any spilled eye-drops, particularly fluorescein.

> Avoid touching the end of the dropper bottle or the nozzle of the tube with your own fingers or on the patient's eyelids or eyelashes. If the tube or bottle is known to be contaminated, it should be discarded and a new bottle or tube brought into use (Qureshi *et al.,* 2006).

Release the eyelid, then ask the patient to close their eye gently and carefully wipe away any surplus fluid. Complete the required documentation.

Teaching patients, parents and relatives to use eye-drops

Ensure that your education for independence includes information on the following:

- Storage of eye-drops at the correct temperature (and not to keep the used bottle for longer than a month).
- Storage of eye-drops safely (not within the reach of children, because like other medicines, their oral effects in overdose can be deadly).
- How to obtain repeat prescriptions (if required).
- What to do if adverse symptoms develop.
- The need for careful hand washing both before and after the procedure.

When teaching parents to instil eye-drops for their children, remember that some children are naturally fearful of having drops instilled into their eyes. It can help to ask the child to lie down with their eyes closed, and pretend to be asleep; they can be told that they are going have some 'raindrops' dropped on to their eyelids. A suitable reward for cooperation (e.g. a sticker on a special chart) may go a long way. Drop two eye-drops into the corner by the inner canthus of the eye to be treated. When the child is asked to open their eyes, a sufficient amount of the eye-drop will roll into the eye for treatment purposes. The excess should be dabbed away and the child cuddled and rewarded. (A similar method was used for a randomised controlled trial by Smith in 1991.)

The key principles of teaching self-instillation of eye-drops are:

- Patients must be knowledgeable about their own condition and treatment (within their personal capabilities).
- If indicated, patients should know how to obtain further supplies of their drops.
- Eye-drops must be stored safely. They are medicines, and some (e.g. atropine) can have fatal consequences if ingested by a small child. They should be stored in accordance with the manufacturer's recommendations.
- Patients must be able to identify the correct eye-drop and the correct frequency of instillation. Help them to establish timings that are easy to remember within the prescription criteria (e.g. breakfast time, lunchtime, teatime, and bedtime). Some departments give patients tick charts to help them remember.
- Patients must wash their hands thoroughly before using eye-drops and should have a box of paper tissues to hand to wipe away excess drops.

Suggest that they sit in a chair which offers good support to their head and neck, and advise them to use the forefinger of the non-dominant hand to gently pull the lower eyelid down to make a little pocket for the eye-drop to go into. Show them how to hold the dropper bottle in their dominant hand, pointing down, between finger and thumb. Show them how to rest the bottle on the forehead and gently squeeze the sides of the bottle until a drop comes out. Explain that if the drop does not land in the lower fornix, they should move the bottle up or down the forehead so that it does.

This is just one way of teaching patients eye-drop instillation. You may know others, but always follow the key principles above. Always try to educate patients for independence, in case their carer is unavailable. Give plenty of encouragement and issue a bottle of artificial teardrops if practice is needed prior to surgery.

For patients who have physical problems instilling their own eye-drops, because they are nervous or have limited arm mobility, there are two devices available on prescription in the UK that can help.

To do ...

Find an up-to-date copy of the British National Formulary and find the section on eye-drops. Check your responsibilities for controlling microbial contamination of eye-drops in the ophthalmic operating theatre, ward and outpatient department.

Application of an eye pad

An eye pad may be applied for the following reasons:

- following an ophthalmic procedure where a retrobulbar, periorbital, subtenon's or subconjunctival injection has been given and the eyelids are not closing satisfactorily
- to promote patient comfort following a deep corneal abrasion
- following eye surgery, either intraocular or to the eyelid.

If you are required to apply an eye pad, there are two key principles to observe. First, if it follows a surgical procedure, it should not be applied so tightly that it causes undue pressure on the eye. Second, every effort should be made to ensure that the eye does not open under the pad, causing the patient to develop a corneal abrasion. An ophthalmologist and the scrub nurse normally apply postoperative eye pads. Usually a small piece of paraffin gauze is gently smoothed over the closed eyelids with gloved hands. This is to inhibit eye opening. A pad and cartella shield are then applied.

This approach can be carried out as a clean procedure if you are required to apply an eye pad in the ophthalmic emergency or outpatient department. Alternatively, instead of applying paraffin gauze, the eyelids can be lightly taped shut using a small strip of surgical tape, and the eye pad firmly applied on top.

A Cochrane Review carried out by Turner and Rabiou (2006) concluded that treating simple corneal abrasions with a patch does not improve healing rates on the first day post injury and does not reduce pain. They recommend that patches are not used for simple corneal abrasions. They do however recommend that further research should focus on the effects of patching large abrasions. As a junior person it will therefore be your responsibility to carry out the ophthalmologist's directions, but when you become entrusted with a personal caseload, you will have to make your own decisions on whether to patch, based on the condition of the patient's eye, the patient's preference and the ophthalmic research available at the time.

Insertion of a 'bandage' corneal lens

Bandage contact lenses are large, soft lenses that do not contain any optical prescription as their use is purely to protect the cornea from perforation, damage, leaking. The lens should be of a high quality, suitable for long term wear, with good oxygen permeability. A large silicone hydrogel lens is suitable, and is inserted on an ophthalmologist's instructions. Reasons for using a 'bandage lens' include:

- treatment of small corneal lacerations
- corneal thinning and danger of perforation
- treatment of large, recalcitrant recurrent erosions
- pain relief of large corneal abrasions.

They may also be used for a pathological problem with the cornea (e.g. bullous keratopathy) or to protect the cornea in severe cases of in-growing eyelashes causing corneal scarring'

You will need:

- a sterile towel on a clean surface (plus a spare sterile towel to protect the patient from any drips)
- a sterile gallipot
- sterile normal saline
- small sterile swabs to dry the eyelids
- a bandage contact lens
- a comfortable treatment chair for the patient
- a good light.

Also have available just in case a minim of oxybuprocaine 0.4 % (Benoxinate™) and a minim of saline 0.9%.

Check the patient's identity and notes to check which eye will require the lens and explain to the patient what you are going to do. Seat them in the chair comfortably, with their head well supported, and the chair adjusted to a good working height. Clean your hands and open the sterile towel (or eye dressing pack) and the minims onto the sterile field. Tip the sterile bandage lens into the gallipot. Wash your hands again (alcohol gel is not recommended at this stage because it could contaminate the bandage lens). Stand behind or facing the patient according to your preference, with your working materials easily accessible to your dominant hand. Put a sterile paper towel around the patient's neck on the affected side.

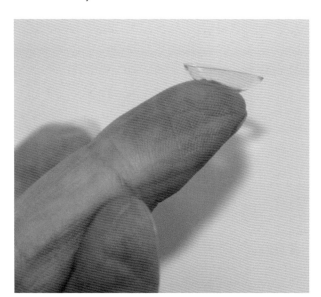

Fig. 14.9

Bandage contact lens ready for insertion

Place the bandage lens on your index finger, then ask your patient to look down. With the first finger of your other hand, pull the upper eyelid fully open, holding it securely, close to the eyelid margin. Then ask the patient to look up, and secure the lower eyelid with your second finger. Being very careful not to drop the lens, gently insert it on to the exposed cornea.

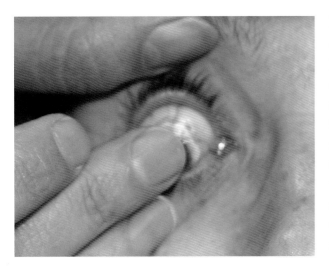

Fig. 14.10
Bandage contact lens applied.

Ensure that the edges are tucked under the eyelids. Ask your patient to blink, and then close their eyelid firmly to remove any air bubbles. When you are learning, you might need to make a second attempt, particularly if the patient has a small eye, or tight lids, or is a 'squeezer'. This is when the oxybuprocaine 0.4% can be useful. If the eye is quite dry, use the saline minim. Make sure that the lens does not get turned 'inside out'.

When instilling eye-drops into a patient's eye where a bandage lens is present, preservative-free drops are normally used (Rubinstein and Evans, 1997).

Ryaz *et al.* (2007) have described a new method for inserting a bandage lens that involves picking up the exterior surface of the lens with the nozzle of a minim by suction, placing it on the cornea and releasing it by breaking the suction. They suggest that it can reduce the risk of infection in already compromised eyes. It is possible that this may prove easier in principle than practice.

Teaching eyelid taping

Lower eyelid taping for entropion relief

Entropion tends to occur in the older people, and is due to dysfunction of the muscle groups in the lower eyelid. Initially it may be unilateral, but it tends to affect both eyes. It is relieved surgically, but at the time of diagnosis the patient may be in considerable discomfort with a lower eyelid that is tending to roll inwards, causing the eyelashes to abrade the cornea. Applying surgical tape is a temporary means of helping the patient to cope while surgery is arranged.

You will need:

- scissors (thoroughly cleaned with a medical wipe prior to use)
- paper surgical tape (e.g. Micropore™ which sticks well and is slightly softer than some other tapes, so if it accidentally detaches it may cause less corneal trauma)
- a mirror for teaching the patient.

Cut a length of paper surgical tape measuring about 26 mm wide. With the entropion of the lower eyelid pulled back into its correct anatomical position, carefully seal the tape on to the skin as close to the lower eyelashes as you can, and gently pull it down, securing the bulk of the tape on the patient's upper cheek. Make sure that your patient (and possibly their carer) knows how to do this. Give the patient a new roll of surgical tape to take home, and ask them to renew the taping as often as required. This is a difficult problem to manage effectively this way, but is worth trying while the patient is waiting for surgery.

Other eyelid problems

You may occasionally be asked to advise a patient who has a condition such as exophthalmos, proptosis or a paralysis of the facial nerve (e.g. Bell's palsy). This might include advice on instilling lubricating eye-drops frequently to prevent corneal exposure. You can also show them how to manually 'blink' their paralysed eyelids by placing a finger on the upper eyelid and moving it up and down.

Sometimes patients are issued with transparent occlusive eye shields to act as 'moisture chambers' and to help prevent dry areas developing on the cornea. A good tip for patients is that if the chamber is 'steaming up', making a tiny pinhole on the periphery of the transparent chamber will alleviate this problem.

Patients also need to be taught how to tape their eyelids closed at night. Cut a length of paper surgical tape (preferably Micropore™) about 13 mm wide. Draw the bottom eyelid up and gently secure paper surgical tape to it. Then, while continuing the gentle traction on the tape holding the lower lid, bring the top eyelid down to meet it using a finger from the other hand. Secure both eyelids shut using the remainder of the tape, leaving a folded over area at the end to facilitate removal of the tape in the morning.

4. MINOR TREATMENTS

Before commencing any treatment, record the history and check and record the central visual acuity. Emergency eye irrigation is the only exception to this rule, and is the procedure that all ophthalmic nurses should be able to carry out without delay. There is a range of ophthalmic procedures undertaken by ophthalmic nurses, and this section is offered as an introduction to some of these.

Eyelid eversion

Reasons for doing this are when:

- you believe there may be something under the top eyelid
- you need to examine the conjunctiva of the upper eyelid
- the person has a chemical injury and you need to thoroughly wash round the eye.

You will need:

- cotton buds moistened with sterile saline
- reading spectacles if you have them
- a good light.

N.B. There are several ways to do this, but this is probably the easiest method when you are learning this skill for the first time.

Wash your hands. Seat your patient in a comfortable chair, with their head well supported. Explain that you are going to look under their top eyelid. Reassure them that what you are about to do will not hurt but may feel rather strange. Ask them to help you by concentrating on looking down. Do not start until you are certain that you feel calm and ready, and your patient feels calm and confident in you. Stand behind the patient, and tilt their head back until it is resting on your chest. Ask them to open both eyes and concentrate on looking down all the time with both eyes. Take a firm hold of the eyelashes of their upper eyelid. Using your other hand, place one end of your cotton bud behind the cartilage plate of the upper eyelid. Push down gently on the cotton bud at the same time as pulling gently the upper eyelashes down and out, away from the eye. Using these movements, gently evert the eyelid, continuously reminding your patient to keep on looking down. Keep holding the eyelid everted with your first three fingers until you have finished your procedure.

Examine the conjunctiva lining the upper eyelid. If you suspect that there may be a foreign body under the top eyelid, use a moist cotton bud to gently remove it. If you cannot see anything, it is wise to gently wipe the inside of the eyelid anyway. Let go of the eyelid and ask your patient to look up. The eyelid will return to its natural position. If you were right, and there was a foreign body under the eyelid, the condition will be immediately improved.

When examining a patient at the slit lamp, you will need to develop the technique of everting the eyelid while the patient is facing you within the restraining frame of the slit lamp. Experienced nurses are able to do this very gently, using just their fingers.

Eye irrigation

Reasons for doing this are:

- to treat acid or alkali burns
- to wash out dust and dirt particles.

You will need:

- a clean, dry work surface
- paper towels and paper tissues
- plastic protection or an apron over the patient's clothing
- a small jug or plastic feeding beaker with lid
- a kidney dish
- a 500 mL sterile normal saline solution at room temperature (an intravenous giving set and normal saline may be used if the irrigation is to be prolonged)
- pH paper
- cotton buds
- local anaesthetic eye-drops
- a Morgan lens (optional).

Waste no time. Check the pH if you are able to do so. Reassure the patient, instil local anaesthetic drops if available, and briefly explain to them what you are going to do, as you get the equipment ready. Protect the patient's clothing with a plastic apron and paper towels. Position them comfortably on their back, on a couch or on a treatment chair, with their head well supported.

Fill the beaker or jug with sterile sodium chloride. Ask them to turn their head slightly towards the affected side. They should hold the kidney dish close to their cheek to catch the irrigation fluid. Hold the lower eyelid down gently and direct the fluid first against the cheek, then inside the bottom eyelid. Ask them to look up, then down, then sideways while the irrigation is continued. Evert the upper eyelid while irrigating underneath it. Dry their eyelids and face prior to the removal of the kidney dish. Remove the plastic apron.

> Remember:
> *Do not record visual acuity first when treating a chemical injury – speed is essential.*

Instil local anaesthetic drops throughout the procedure as necessary, as these are being constantly leeched out by the irrigation process. Use a Desmarres retractor to double evert the upper eyelid if necessary. If you do not have one, improvise with moistened cotton buds.

Remove any solid material with a wet cotton bud. You may require a fine pair of forceps (such as Mathelone's) to remove material that is wedged in the conjunctival surface. Fluid should not be directed on to the eye from a distance of greater than about 4 cm. Irrigation must be continued until the pH is back to normal. Expect that severe chemical burns may require slow irrigation for up to an hour, using an intravenous giving set, with possibly a Morgan lens if you have one available. It may be possible to move the patient's couch up to the sink, and support their head over the sink for this treatment.

Check and record visual acuity before a doctor sees the patient. Continue irrigating as necessary.

Concretion removal

'Concretions' are creamy white inclusion cysts filled with keratin and epithelial debris that are found in the palpaebral conjunctiva of the upper and lower eyelids. They are completely benign. However, occasionally a patient complains of a scratchy sensation and on examination it may be seen that one of these deposits is sticking through the conjunctiva and scratching the front of the eye. Any troublesome concretion can be easily and painlessly removed, but you should only do this under the guidance of an experienced ophthalmic nurse or doctor until your competency has been officially recognised within your department.

You can read more about this condition in Austen (1999) and the Handbook of Ocular Disease Management online.

You will need:

- local anaesthetic eye-drops
- a slit lamp or magnifying loupe headband
- an injection needle of an appropriate size
- a syringe (1mL) to mount the injection needle on
- cotton swabs
- cotton-wool buds, moistened at the tip with a drop from the local anaesthetic minim.

Explain to your patient what you are going to do and why. Instil a local anaesthetic eye-drop in the area of the concretion and wait for 3 minutes for it to work. Prepare your equipment out of the patient's direct line of sight. Mention the use of 'a small instrument' and the importance of the patient keeping very still for a few moments. Use the side of the injection needle like a sharp-sided spoon to scoop and lift out the concretion. Sometimes you may need the moistened swab to 'capture' crumbs from the concretion. There is sometimes a little bleeding following removal, particularly if the patient is taking aspirin or warfarin. A little gentle pressure can be applied to the bleeding area with a moistened cotton bud. No routine after care is required for this small procedure.

You will need to have undergone supervised practice and demonstrate sufficient knowledge and consistently satisfactory practice before you are accredited to carry out this procedure unsupervised.

Epilation of an eyelash

Eyelashes that are abrading the cornea need to be carefully evaluated. If the eyelash can readily be brushed back into the normal position, and if the patient following advice can maintain it in the normal position, it should not be removed. Removal could cause it to grow back at a slightly different, less advantageous angle.

These days epilation of eyelashes normally takes place with the patient positioned at the slit lamp. Pull the eyelid slightly away from the eye with a finger. A good pair of forceps such as Mathelone's or jeweller's forceps is necessary to grasp the eyelash securely, as close to its base as possible. With a tight grip around the lash, ensure that the patient's cornea is tilted away from your forceps, and maintaining a steady pressure, pull the eyelash out in the direction of its growth.

Check the cornea for any abrasions caused by the lash rubbing, and treat accordingly. As the eyelash follicles stay intact, there will be re-growth, and the patient needs advice regarding re-treatment.

To do ...

Find out about trichiasis and distichiasis.

Removal of a superficial corneal foreign body

If a foreign body is lying on the cornea, it is likely to cause damage to the delicate endothelial surface of the cornea. Poking at it may cause damage, so in the first instance it is a good plan to see if the debris can be floated off the cornea by flushing it with a minim of normal saline. If it is displaced into the lower fornix, it can be very safely removed by asking the patient to look up, to tilt the cornea out of the way, and then removing it with a slightly moist cotton bud.

If flushing the corneal foreign body with sterile normal saline fails to remove it, but it is not embedded, it may be possible to remove it by instilling a local anaesthetic eye-drop. When the drop has had time to take effect, try gently brushing the foreign body with a moist cotton bud to remove it. Do not use any force, as no matter how gentle you are, you will still cause a slight corneal abrasion. Trained, experienced ophthalmic staff carry out the procedure below.

You will need:

- anaesthetic drops (e.g. proxyametacaine hydrochloride 0.5% (Ophthaine™), oxybuprocaine hydrochloride 0.4% (Benoxinate™)
- a No. 1 disposable injection needle
- cotton-wool buds
- the patient's notes.

Wash your hands. Examine both eyes. Explain to the patient what you are going to do, ensure they are positioned comfortably at the slit lamp. Anaesthetise the affected eye with the local anaesthetic eye-drops. Ask the patient to keep both eyes open and to focus on a distant object. Ensure that the patient's forehead is firmly pressed against the top headband of the slit lamp throughout the procedure. This is for two good reasons – if they move back, they go out of slit lamp focus, and with the head kept firmly on the band they cannot move forwards on to your needle, they can only move away. Holding the injection needle horizontally and tangentially to the cornea, gently lift the foreign body off the cornea.

It may be necessary, depending on the location of the foreign body and whether the patient is able to keep his eye open, to hold the upper and lower lids of the affected eye open with your 'spare' hand. This of course, can make it difficult to keep the slit lamp in focus.

Record all your findings and treatment. If required, antibiotic eye-drops may be supplied according to local protocols. The patient should be asked to return to the eye department for further examination or treatment if required.

> This procedure should only be carried under supervision until your competence and experience has been assessed.

Conclusion

The nurse or professional allied to medicine (PAM) should always aim to give care that is of the highest quality. Ophthalmic nurses and optometrists have developed a wide range of published specialised knowledge and research. The ophthalmic patient needs to remain the focus of our care, beyond our own needs for experience and knowledge acquisition, and must be treated with respect as regards their personal fears, frailty and needs. With this in mind, the Ophthalmic Nursing Forum (2009) has re-issued their publication *The Nature, Scope and Value of Ophthalmic Nursing* to remind us of our therapeutic relationship with patients, as well as the importance of two-way communication between the patient and professional and the significance of patient education. This document identifies nine key standards of care, together with the means to audit these, and is essential reading for all who work within the field of ophthalmic care.

References and further reading

Austen, P. (1999). Conjunctival concretion removal. *Optometry Today*. September 24, 33–34. Available at: http://www.otmagazine.co.uk/articles.php?year = 1999 (last accessed August 2009).

Benner, P. (1984). *From Novice to Expert*. Reading, USA: Addison Wesley.

Bitsios, P., Prettyman, R. and Szabadi, E. (1996). Changes in autonomic function with age: a study of pupillary kinetics in healthy young and old people. *Age and Ageing*, 25(6), 432–38.

Cagle, G. and Abshire, R. (1981). Quantitative ocular bacteriology for the enumeration and identification of bacteria from the skin lash margin and conjunctiva. *Investigative Ophthalmology and Visual Science*, 20, 753–58.

Casser, C., Fingeret, M. and Woodcombe, H. (1997). *Atlas of Primary Eye Care Procedures*, 2nd edn. New York: McGraw Hill.

Chern, K., Foley, E., Koo, J., Reddy, A. and Sandoval, B. (2004). *Ophthalmic Office Procedures*. New York: McGraw Hill.

Crossland, M. and Rubin, G. (2007). The Amsler chart: Absence of evidence is not evidence of absence. *British Journal of Ophthalmology*, 91(3), 391–93.

Curtis, C., Lo, E., Ooi, L. and Bennett, L. (2009). Factors affecting compliance with eye-drop therapy for glaucoma in a multicultural outpatient setting. *Contemporary Nurse*, 12, 128.

Driver and Vehicle Licensing Agency (2009). *At-a-glance guide to the current medical standards of fitness to drive*. Swansea: Drivers Medical Group, DVLA. Available at: http://www.dvla.gov.uk/medical/ataglance.aspx (last accessed August 2009).

Field, D. and Tillotson, J. (2008). *Eye Emergencies, The Practitioner's Guide*. Keswick: M&K Update.

Hawksworth, N. (2008). *Ophthalmic Instrument Decontamination*. London: Royal College of Ophthalmologists.

Hazel, C. and Elliott, D. (2002). The dependency of logMAR visual acuity measurements on chart design and scoring rule. *Optometry and Visual Science*, 79(12), 788–92.

Health and Safety Executive (2005). *Colour vision examination. A guide for occupational health providers, Note MS7*. 3rd edn. Available at: http://www.hse.gov.uk/pubns/ms7.pdf (last accessed August 2009).

Hillier, R. and Kumar, N. (2008). Tonometer disinfection practice in the United Kingdom: a national survey. *Eye*, 22(8), 1029–33.

Hussain, B., Saleh, G., Sivaprasad, G. and Hammond, C. (2006). Changing from Snellen to logMAR – Debate or delay? *Clinical and Experimental Ophthalmology*, 34(1), 6–8.

Kanski, J, (2007). *Clinical Ophthalmology*. Oxford: Butterworth Heinemann.

Lim, R., Dhillon, B., Kurian, K., Aspinall, P., Fernie, K. and Ironside, J. (2003). Retention of corneal epithelial cells following Goldman applanation tonometry: implications for CJD risk. *British Journal of Ophthalmology*, 87(5), 583–6.

Macdonald, M. and Ramasethu, J. (2007). *Atlas of Procedures in Neonatology*, 4th edn. Philadelphia: Lippincott, Williams and Wilkins.

Maino, A., Morgan, L., Hercules, B. and Tullo, A. (2006a). Ophthalmology, Are disposable prisms an adequate alternative to standard Goldmann tonometry prisms in glaucoma patients? *Ophthalmology*, 113(10), 1837–41.

Maino, A., Uddin, H. and Tullo, A. (2006b). A comparison of the clinical performance between disposable and Goldman tonometers. *Eye*, 20(5), 574–78.

Moutray, T., Williams, M. and Jackson, A. (2008). Change of visual acuity recording methods in clinical studies across the years. *Ophthalmologica*, 222, 173–77.

Mullin, G. and Rubinfeld, R. (1997). The antibacterial activity of topical anaesthesia. *Cornea*, 16, 662–65.

Nayak, N. and Satpathy, G. (2000). Slime production as a virulence factor in Staphylococcus epidermidis isolated from bacterial keratitis. *Indian Journal of Medical Research*, 55, 9–13.

Ophthalmic Nursing Forum (2009). *The nature, scope and value of ophthalmic nursing*. London: Royal College of Nursing. Available at: http://www.rcn.org.uk/development/publications/search?mode = publications&q_title = Nature + Scope + Value + Ophthalmic + Nursing&logic_title = AND (last accessed August 2009).

Qureshi, M., Wong, S., Robbie, K., Qureshi, C. and Rowe, J. (2006). Contamination of single use minims eye-drops by multiple use in clinics. *Journal of Hospital Infection*, 62(2), 245–47.

Rajak, J., Paul, J., Sharma, V. and Vickers, S. (2006). Contamination of disposable prisms during applanation tonometry. *Eye*, 20(3), 388.

Redmond, N. and While, A. (2008). Dry eye syndrome and watering eye. *British Journal of Community Nursing*, 13(10), 471–79.

Reid, L. (2006). *Functional assessment of vision*. Scottish Sensory Centre. Available at: http://www.ssc.education.ed.ac.uk/courses/vi&multi/vmay06a.html (last accessed August 2009).

Rose, K. (2000). Vision testing in the outpatients' department. *Ophthalmic Nursing*, 4(3), 24–26.

Rose. K., Waterman, H. and Tullo, A. (1997). A qualitative analysis of loss of vision due to cataract. *Ophthalmic Nursing,* 1, 4–10.

Rubinstein, M. and Evans, J. (1997). Therapeutic contact lenses and eye-drops – is there a problem? *Contact Lens and the Anterior Eye,* 20(1), 9–11.

Ryaz, A., Manjunatha, N. and Desai, S. (2007). Insertion of a bandage contact lens with minims. *Eye and Contact Lens: Science and Clinical Practice,* 33(2), 89–90.

Sandhu, S., Chattopadhyay, S., Birch, M. and Ray-Chaudhuri, N. (2005). Frequency of Goldman applanation tonometer calibration error checks. *Journal of Glaucoma,* 14(3), 215–18.

Sheridan, M. and Gardiner, P. (1970). Sheridan–Gardiner test for visual acuity. *British Medical Journal,* 2(5701), 108–09.

Skorin, L. (2002). Eyelid misdirection and it is management. *Optometry Magazine,* September 20. Available at: http://www.optometry.co.uk/articles/docs/70cde392b25e1d895b6405016e56d892_skorin20020920.pdf (last accessed October 2009).

Smith, S. (1991). Eye-drop instillation for reluctant children. *British Journal of Ophthalmology,* 75(8), 480–81.

Sobol, A. (2007). *Seidel test animation.* Available at: http://drsobol.com/Default.aspx?blogentryid = 36 (last accessed August 2009).

Tattersall, C. (2006). Improving the accuracy of intraocular pressure readings. *Nursing Times,* 102(27), 36–38.

Thomson, D. (2005). Visual acuity testing in optometric practice. Part 2: Newer chart designs. *Optometry Today,* May 6. Available at: http://www.optometry.co.uk/articles.php?year = 2005 (last accessed August 2009).

Turner, A. and Rabiou, M. (2006). Patching for corneal abrasion. *Cochrane Database Systemic Review,* April 19 (2), CD 004764.

Watkinson, S. and Seewoodhary, R. (2008). Administering eye medications. *Nursing Standard,* 22(18), 42–48.

Witchell, L. (1998). Measuring intra-ocular pressure. *International Journal of Ophthalmic Nursing,* 4(1), 22–25.

Wolfel, R., Pfeffer, M., Esbauer, S., Nerkelun, S. and Dobler, G. (2006). Evaluation of sampling technique and transport media for the diagnostics of adenoviral eye infections. *Graefe's Archive for Clinical and Experimental Ophthalmology* 244(11), 487–504.

Useful web resources

Colorblind
http://colorvisiontesting.com/
T. Waggoner's site about colour blindness.

Handbook of Ocular Disease Management
http://www.revoptom.com/HANDBOOK/hbhome.htm
For information on conjunctival concretions.

Health Professions Council Standards of Proficiency
http://www.hpc-uk.org/

Look Up
http://www.lookupinfo.org/
Information on eye care and vision for people with learning disabilities. Check the 'eye care' section for excellent information on helping people with learning difficulties deal with eye-drops.

National Eye Institute
http://www.nei.nih.gov/
Look for the Early Treatment Diabetic Retinopathy Study (ETDS).

National Glaucoma Society (USA)
http://www.nationalglaucomasociety.org/

Nursing and Midwifery Council
http://www.nmc-uk.org/
This includes the Code of Professional Conduct 2008.

Opticare (eye-drop devices)
http://www.opticare.org.uk/

The Eye Digest
http://www.ageingeye.net/dryeyes/dryeyeseyeexam.php
The dry eye examination.

Thomson Software Solutions
http://www.thomson-software-solutions.com/
Software for eye care.

Record of ophthalmic knowledge and skills development

This section is to give you, as an ophthalmic professional, some personal evidence of your developing proficiency and to help you identify any gaps in your personal experience. The document is arranged in five key areas:

1. Ophthalmic tests and investigations.

2. Eye care.

3. Minor interventions.

4. Equipment use.

5. Ophthalmic theatres.

An additional continuation sheet is also provided and there is space within each section for you to add extra information. Remember that equipment, responsibilities and practices will keep changing. You can use the blank spaces and the continuation sheet to record them. The ophthalmic theatre record has been left blank so that you can enter information that specifically reflects your personal professional responsibilities. It is expected that there will be some 'cross over' of certain responsibilities into other areas, and activities in some areas may 'cross over' into theatre experiences.

Do not be frightened at the number of areas listed here. It is unlikely that you will be able to cover all of them as the complexity of modern ophthalmology often results in people specialising in specific areas.

All practice should be carried out in accordance with the Nursing and Midwifery Council's Code of Conduct 2008 or the Health Professions Council Standards of Proficiency. Proficiency in practice (Benner, 1984) denotes more than mere task completion, as the proficient person will perceive and understand situations as wholes rather than as isolated incidents or encounters. The patient is seen in terms of their past, present and future. Any skilled intervention is guided by professional standards, experience and research or academic knowledge as well as psychomotor skill performance. The proficient professional is beginning to sense nuances within the practice situation, acting in anticipation of potential needs or changes of circumstance.

How to record the information

To fill in the records – which must avoid the old 'see one, do one, kill one' approach – you must first obtain instruction in the procedure, via practical demonstration (either in a classroom as part of an eye course or in clinical practice) and this should be dated and signed by the instructor, who might be your mentor or another senior ophthalmic professional.

At a later date, you will be observed performing the procedure under supervision in clinical practice and again this must be signed and dated.

Finally, at a later date, when consistent, fully competent practice and problem solving has been observed and assessed by interview, you will be signed off as proficient.

Remember, this documentation is yours – make it work to assist your development. It can also be used as evidence at your annual appraisal or to provide underpinning credibility of your experience at a job interview.

1. Ophthalmic tests and investigations

Test/investigation	Instruction (date/sign)	Practice (date/sign)	Proficient (date/sign)
Snellen vision test			
LogMAR test			
Sheridan–Gardiner test			
Near vision test			
Ishihara colour vision test			
Amsler grid			
Conjunctival swabs for culture			
Lacrimal sac syringing			
Schirmer's test			
Goldman applanation tonometry			
Seidel's test			
Pupil reactions			

2. Eye care

Procedure	Instruction (date/sign)	Practice (date/sign)	Proficient (date/sign)
Cleaning a patient's eyelids			
Eye-drop and ointment instillation			
Application of an eye pad			
Insertion of a bandage contact lens			
Teaching eyelid taping			
Postoperative management of the eye socket			
Insertion of a shell			
Removal and re-insertion of an artificial eye			

3. Minor interventions

Intervention	Instruction (date/sign)	Practice (date/sign)	Proficient (date/sign)
Eyelid eversion			
Eye irrigation			
Removal of concretions			
Removal of a superficial foreign body			
Epilation of eyelashes			
Ophthalmic suture removal			

4. Equipment use

Equipment	Instruction (date/sign)	Practice (date/sign)	Proficient (date/sign)
Slit lamp			
TonoPen™			
Autorefractor			
Keratometer			
Focimeter			
A-Scan (manual biometry)			
IOL Master™			
Automated field analyzer (Humphrey)			
Visual field interpretation			
Optical coherence tomography (OTC) imaging			
Heidelberg retinal tomogram (HRT) imaging			
Use of trial lenses			

5. Ophthalmic theatres

	Instruction (date/sign)	Practice (date/sign)	Proficient (date/sign)

6. Continuation sheet

	Instruction (date/sign)	Practice (date/sign)	Proficient (date/sign)

6. Continuation sheet

Glossary of common ophthalmic abbreviations, acronyms and terms

a/c see Anterior chamber

Acanthamoeba keratitis An infection of the cornea by a tiny amoeba organism, often caused by washing contact lenses in infected water, followed by poor contact lens hygiene.

Accommodation The ability of the lens to alter its thickness and allow objects to be focused on the retina.

Afferent pupillary defect A nerve pathway from one of the eyes fails to transmit a message to the brain.

Akinesia A general term which, within ophthalmology, relates to an inability to move the eye or squeeze the eyelids shut.

Amaurosis fugax A sudden, transient loss of vision affecting only one eye.

Amblyopic eye A normal eye that does not see clearly even with spectacles (often caused by an inadequately treated squint in childhood).

AMD Age-related macular degeneration. Sometimes known as ARMD.

Anaesthetic cornea Loss of sensation in the cornea, often as a result of viral keratitis. The condition is said to be potentially blinding as it can mean that major infection and trauma to the cornea are not detected.

Aniridia A congenitally incomplete iris.

Anisocoria Unequal pupil size.

Anophthalmos Failure of the eye to develop during early pregnancy. The child may be born with no eyes at all, or with vestigial eyes.

Anterior chamber The space between the anterior surface of the iris and the posterior (endothelial) surface of the cornea.

Anterior segment of the eye This comprises the anterior and posterior chambers.

Aphakia An eye from which the lens has been removed.

Aqueous humour The transparent fluid that fills the anterior chamber of the eye.

Astigmatism An irregular shape to the front of the cornea. Without spectacle correction, this may cause a varying degree of visual distortion.

BDR Background diabetic retinopathy.

BE Both eyes.

Bifocal spectacles Spectacles with clearly defined areas for distant and near vision.

Binocular vision The ability of both eyes to focus on an object and to fuse the two images into a single image.

Blepharitis Inflammation of the eyelid margins.

Blepharospasm A sustained involuntary spasm of the muscles controlling the eyelids, causing them to be squeezed shut.

Blind spot A blind area in the visual field that corresponds to the position of the head of the optic nerve.

Blow-out fracture A fracture of the orbital floor in which some of the orbital contents prolapse into the maxillary sinus.

Branch vein occlusion Occlusion of a branch of the central retinal vein.

BRAO Branch retinal artery occlusion.

BRVO Branch retinal vein occlusion.

Bullous keratopathy This occurs as a result of deterioration of the number and efficiency of corneal endothelial cells. The remaining 'pump cells' are unable to maintain normal corneal hydration. The cornea becomes waterlogged and excess fluid forms blisters under the corneal epithelium. When these bullae (blisters) burst, corneal nerves are exposed and the eye becomes acutely painful.

Canal of Schlemm A circular drainage canal situated at the limbus for draining aqueous fluid from the anterior chamber.

Canthus The inner and outer 'corners' of the eye (properly described as the lateral canthus and the medial canthus).

Capsulorhexis A circular tear made in the anterior lens capsule during cataract surgery.

Carotid bruit An abnormal sound heard by stethoscope applied to the carotid artery, indicating partial occlusion of the artery.

Cartella shield A plastic shield with perforations (usually clear) that is used to protect the eye.

Caruncle The fleshy lump at the inner corner of the eye.

Cataract An opacity of the normally transparent lens.

Central retinal artery occlusion (CRAO) Occlusion of the central retinal artery.

Central retinal vein occlusion (CRVO) Occlusion of the central retinal vein.

Chalazion This is often referred to as a meibomian cyst, as it is a granulomatous inflammation of a meibomian gland.

Chemosis Swelling of the conjunctiva.

Chiasma (optic) A chiasma is a cross-over point. At the optic chiasma some of the nerve fibres from each eye cross over, and are directed to the opposite side of the brain for visual interpretation.

Ciliary flush A circle of tiny dilated blood vessels around the corneal periphery.

Coloboma A gap in a body tissue caused by an incomplete development process. Within ophthalmology a simple coloboma may be seen in the eyelid or the iris. More seriously it can involve the choroid, lens, optic nerve or disc. Other areas of the body may also be involved.

Concretion Cream coloured inclusion cysts inside the upper or lower eyelids filled with keratin and epithelial debris.

Conjunctival cyst A small, fluid-filled cyst arising from the conjunctiva either inside the eyelid or from the bulbar conjunctiva covering the sclera.

Conjunctivitis An inflammation of the conjunctiva in response to an infection (bacterial or viral), allergy or irritant.

Corneal dystrophies A range of rare conditions of the cornea that affect different layers of the cornea.

Corneal graft Use of a donor cornea to replace a damaged or diseased cornea. Grafts can be full-thickness or lamellar (partial thickness).

Corneal ulcer Damage caused to the surface of the cornea as a direct result of infection, or indirectly from an infected injury.

CRAO Central retinal artery occlusion.

C-reactive protein test A measure of the concentration of a protein in the blood serum that indicates inflammation.

CRVO Central retinal vein occlusion.

Cycloplegia Paralysis of the ciliary muscle, causing the lens to flatten, as if focusing for distance vision.

D see Dioptre

Dacryocystectomy Excision of the nasolacrimal sac.

Dacryocystitis Infection and inflammation of the nasolacrimal sac.

Dacryocystorhinostomy A procedure to create a new passage for a blocked nasolacrimal duct.

Dendritic ulcer A corneal ulcer with a typically branched appearance, resulting from a herpes simplex or herpes zoster infection.

Descemetocele A bulging area of Descemet's membrane caused by damage to the corneal surface.

Diabetic retinopathy Changes in the visible characteristics of the blood vessels of the retina.

Dioptre A unit used in prescribing lenses. 1 dioptre (+ or –) will adjust a person's focus by 1 metre.

Diplopia Double vision.

Distance glasses Spectacle lenses for driving and watching television, etc.

Distichiasis Abnormal growth of an extra band of eyelashes from the orifices of the meibomian glands. These eyelashes lie across the front surface of the eye.

Drusen Creamy yellow deposits visible on the retina, arising from Bruch's membrane. They are often benign, but when they appear in the macular area they may be associated with age-related macular degeneration.

Dystrophy A congenital condition that may be initially asymptomatic.

Ectropion A 'loose' lower eyelid that does not maintain good contact with the eye.

Endophthalmitis A severe infection affecting the internal structures of the eyeball.

Enophthalmos An eye that looks smaller than its fellow, as a result of a fracture to the orbital floor or developmental defect.

Entropion A 'tight' lower eyelid that tends to roll inwards causing the eyelashes to abrade the cornea.

Enucleation Removal of the eye.

Epilation Removal of an eyelash.

Epiphora Excessive watering of an eye.

Evisceration Removal of the contents of the eye, leaving the extraocular muscles and sclera within the orbit.

Exenteration Radical surgery for an invasive tumour of the orbit or surrounding skin. The contents of the orbit are removed, but the eyelids are sometimes spared, depending on the location of the tumour.

Exophthalmos One or both eyes protrudes outwards. It is often associated with thyroid over-activity.

Flare Protein in the aqueous fluid as a product of anterior uveitis. It is seen in a narrow slit lamp beam as a result of its light-scattering properties.

Floaters Debris in the vitreous. Described by patients as spots or spiders occurring in the field of vision.

FOH Family ophthalmic history.

Follicles Raised, rounded, avascular white or grey structures containing lymphocytes that are found in the conjunctiva lining the lower eyelid and the border of the upper tarsal plate. They are frequently noted in viral and chlamydial infections or with allergies to eye medications.

Fornix (fornices) Pouches under the upper and lower eyelids. They are formed by the conjunctiva covering the inside of the eyelids folding back on itself to cover the anterior surface of the eye.

Fovea The structure lying at the centre of the macula which is responsible for the sharpest vision.

Fundus The area that can be seen through an ophthalmoscope which includes the macula, optic disc, optic nerve and central retinal artery and vein.

g. Guttae (eye-drops).

Geographic ulcer Associated with corneal infection with herpes simplex. Misdiagnosis resulting in inappropriate steroid treatment can result in a lesion becoming a geographic corneal ulcer.

Giant cell arteritis Another name for temporal arteritis.

Glaucoma A collective term for a number of eye conditions generally – not invariably associated with raised intraocular pressure.

Gonioscope A contact lens containing a mirror or mirrors, used with the slit lamp to examine the trabecular meshwork.

Hemianopia Loss of half of the visual field in one or both eyes.

Herpes simplex Infection with herpes simplex type 1 causes cold sores and can cause corneal ulcers. Many people have this virus, which lies dormant between attacks, but occasionally becomes re-activated.

Herpes zoster ophthalmicus (HZO) This is caused by the varicella zoster virus which is generally acquired in childhood as chickenpox. It remains dormant in the body and on re-activation it causes 'shingles', in this instance affecting the area supplied by the ophthalmic division of the trigeminal nerve.

HMs Hand movements.

Hordeolum An external hordeolum is a stye. An internal hordeolum is a meibomian cyst.

Hutchinson's sign If the rash in herpes zoster ophthalmicus reaches down the side of the nose to the nasal tip, the patient is more likely to have corneal involvement in the infection process.

Hypermetropia This is 'long-sightedness" whereby the person sees better at a distance than near, due to a shorter than average eyeball.

Hyphaema Blood present in the anterior chamber of the eye.

Hypopion A mass of white inflammatory cells in the anterior chamber of the eye.

Intraocular pressure The hydrostatic pressure inside the eye.

IOL Intraocular lens.

IOP see Intraocular pressure

Iridectomy Removal of part of the iris.

K As in K readings with a keratometer to measure the corneal curvature.

Keratic precipitates Groups of inflammatory cells adhering to the posterior surface of the cornea.

Keratitis Inflammation of the cornea.

Keratoconus A progressive degenerative disorder of the cornea, generally noted at puberty, which causes the cornea to become conical in shape.

Keratoplasty Alternative name for a corneal graft.

KPs see Keratic precipitates

Lacrimation Excessive watering of the eye.

Lagophthalmos An inability to adequately close the upper eyelid.

LASIK Laser-assisted in situ keratomileusis. Otherwise known as laser refractive surgery.

Lazy eye A normal eye which was at some stage misaligned. The brain never received a clear image on this side, and visual perception via the optic nerves and brain did not develop as well as it might have done.

LE Left eye.

Limbus This is a transitional area where the cornea and sclera meet.

LTG Low-tension glaucoma.

LVA Low visual aid (e.g. a magnifying glass).

Marfan syndrome A widespread disease of connective tissue associated with cardiac abnormalities, skeletal anomalies and muscular underdevelopment. Ophthalmically, these people are prone to lens dislocation and glaucoma.

Meibomian cyst A cyst in the eyelid caused by a blocked meibomian gland.

Meibomianitis Inflammation of the meibomian glands in the eyelids.

Microphthalmos A small eye that does not function normally and may have other congenital abnormalities (e.g. of the lens).

Micropsia A perceptual reduction in the size of objects viewed with the affected eye. This indicates serious macular pathology.

Minim A volume approximating the size of one drop. In ophthalmology this refers to a tiny container of eye-drops intended for a single use.

Miotic A drug that constricts the pupil.

Moll (cyst of) A small, pearly looking fluid-filled cyst on the eyelid margin, arising from a gland of Moll at the base of an eyelash.

Monocular diplopia Double vision perceived by only one eye. It may be a symptom of cataract.

Mydriatic A drug that dilates the pupil.

Myopia This is 'short sightedness' whereby the person's near vision is better than their distant vision.

Nanophthalmos A condition where both eyes are congenitally abnormally small.

Neovascularisation The development of abnormal new blood vessels. In the eye this may occur initially at the retina as a result of retinal ischaemia. Unchecked, new vessels may grow forward over the iris and into the drainage angle.

NPL No perception of light.

NTG Normal tension glaucoma.

Nystagmus Uncontrolled, generally sideways movements of the eyes associated with very poor vision.

Occ. Occulentum (the Latin word for ointment).

Ocular albinos A pigmentation disorder of the eye. People with this have skin and hair pigmentation like that of their other family members, but their eyes are lacking in melanin. Vision is poor because large amounts of light are able to enter the eye, and the iris is not an effective shield without its pigment layer. The retina's pigment layer is not present to absorb light.

Ophthalmia neonatorum Also known as neonatal conjunctivitis. This is defined as any purulent discharge from the eyes of a newborn baby within 14 days of birth. It is a notifiable disease.

Ophthalmologist A qualified doctor who holds post-registration qualifications in ophthalmology or who is undertaking studies in this field.

Ophthalmoscope An instrument for examining the vitreous, retina or optic disc. It may be a 'direct ophthalmoscope' that is held directly to the examiner's eye, or an 'indirect ophthalmoscope' that shines a beam of light from a band on the examiner's head through a magnifying glass and into the patient's eye, producing an inverted view of the retina (the latter is better for examining the periphery of the retina).

Optic disc At the back of the eye the sclera is pierced by the optic nerve, central retinal artery and central retinal vein. It appears as a slightly depressed area, and contains no rods or cones, and is therefore the 'blind spot' of the eye. An abnormally pale or 'cupped' disc is an indicator of primary open-angle glaucoma.

Orbital cellulitis An infection of the soft tissues lying within the orbit.

Orthoptic department Put literally 'orthoptic' means 'straight eyes'. This department concentrates on diagnosing, treating and advising on disorders of vision and defects of eye movements.

p/c *see Posterior chamber*

Pachymeter An instrument used to undertake pachymetry (measurement of corneal thickness).

Palpaebral Relating to the eyelids.

Papillae Tiny raised structures seen within the eyelids, filled with vascular cores. They are a non-specific sign of conjunctival inflammation.

Papilloedema A swollen optic disc with blurred edges and dilated superficial capillaries.

PDT Photodynamic therapy.

Peripheral vision The ability to perceive objects at the side when looking straight ahead.

PERLA An acronym for 'pupils equal and reacting to light and accommodation'.

PH Pin hole.

Photokeratitis The medical term for 'arc eye' or 'welding flash'.

Photophobia Sensitivity to light.

Photopsia 'Flashing lights' perceived in response to an abnormal pull on the retina from shrinking vitreous.

Pingueculum (plural pinguecula) Small, round, yellowish lumps appearing on the conjunctiva on either side of the cornea at 9 o'clock and 3 o'clock positions. They are the result of corneal degeneration, and are benign.

POAG Primary open-angle glaucoma.

Posterior chamber The aqueous-filled space behind the iris and in front of the lens.

Posterior segment The vitreous cavity.

Presbyopia The loss of accommodation of the lens, which becomes hardened due to ageing.

Proptosis Protrusion of one or both eyes.

Pseudophakic An aphakic eye with a lens implant.

Pterygium A superficial, fleshy, vascular wing of conjunctiva, which slowly extends on to the cornea, and may eventually cover the pupillary area.

Ptosis A drooping upper eyelid.

PVD Posterior vitreous detachment.

RAPD Relative afferent pupillary defect.

RD see Retinal detachment

RE Right eye.

Reading glasses Used to correct presbyopia. Unsuitable to use when attempting to read the Snellen chart.

Red desaturation A visual symptom that occurs in optic nerve disease (e.g. optic neuritis).

Red reflex A red light reflected back from the retina when a bright light is shone into the eye. Normal eyes do this, as typically seen in coloured flash photographs. Absence of the red reflex is usually associated with serious retinal pathology.

Refractive error Light rays entering the eye do not focus on the retina.

Retinal detachment Separation of the neural layers of the retina from the pigment epithelium.

Retinitis pigmentosa A hereditary eye disorder accompanied by difficulty in seeing in poor lighting conditions, poor colour vision and progressively deteriorating near and peripheral vision.

Retinoblastoma A rare cancer of the retina, occurring in children, which can be familial. Children often present with a 'white pupil'. If not treated urgently and effectively, the condition can be fatal.

Retinopathy of prematurity A bilateral retinal problem of premature babies born at less than 36 weeks' gestation, or of very low birth weight, weighing less than about 3lb 3oz (1.45 kg) at birth.

Rods and cones The photoreceptors of the retina.

RP see Retinitis pigmentosa

Scotoma A visual field defect.

Sjogren syndrome An autoimmune disorder involving the lacrimal and salivary glands (dry eyes and mouth) and potentially many other areas of the body. It occurs most frequently in women and is frequently associated with rheumatic disorders.

Steroid responder A person whose intraocular pressure rises after the use of steroid eye-drops.

Superficial punctate keratitis (SPKs) Tiny, diffuse corneal lesions with many varied causes (e.g. dry eye, severe conjunctivitis, ultraviolet light exposure or chemical splash).

Sympathetic ophthalmitis An inflammation occurring in the 'good' eye following a severe injury to the 'exciting' eye; it may have occurred days, months or even years previously. Without treatment the 'sympathising' eye may go blind.

Synaechiae These may be anterior (the iris may become adherent to areas of the drainage angle due to lying in prolonged apposition to it) or posterior (there is adhesion of the lens to the iris, again as a result of prolonged contact or due to an inflammatory condition).

Tarsorrhaphy The suturing together partially or completely of the eyelids, generally to cover and heal a corneal ulcer.

Tonometer An instrument used for measuring the intraocular pressure.

Toxacaris A nematode worm that infects dogs or cats and can be acquired by humans. The worm migrates to the human eye where it dies and sets up an extreme inflammatory reaction.

Trichiasis Eyelashes that grow unevenly, usually in response to chronic eyelid inflammation.

VA Visual acuity.

Varifocal spectacles Spectacles that work on a similar principle to bifocals, but without a hard line between the distance and near sections of the lens. The lenses slowly merge, providing some correction for the intermediate distance.

VEGF Vascular endothelial growth factor. It is produced by the body's cells to stimulate new blood vessel formation throughout the body. It is currently of particular interest in ophthalmology as new treatments are being sought for conditions like diabetic retinopathy and age-related macular degeneration

Zeiss (cyst of) A yellow fluid-filled cyst on the eyelid margin that arises from a blocked gland of Zeiss.

Answers to Self Tests

Chapter 2
Basic anatomy and physiology of the eye

1. Check this with the diagram of the eye in Fig. 2.1.
2. The upper punctum and the lower punctum.
3. In the lacrimal gland.
4. It enables the tear film to be held on the front of the eye.
5. The aqueous layer of the basal tear film.
6. It controls the hydration of the cornea by pumping excess fluid back into the aqueous.
7. The iris, ciliary body and choroid.
8. The sphincter pupillae and the dilator pupillae.
9. To focus the lens and secrete aqueous humour.
10. Progressive difficulty focusing the lens of the eye for near vision associated with ageing.
11. The trabecular meshwork, the canal of Schlemm and the episcleral/conjunctival veins.
12. The uveoscleral route.
13. The neural layer and the pigment layer.
14. The optic disc, optic nerve, the central retinal artery and the macula.
15. Colour vision.
16. The optic chiasma.

Chapter 3
Basic refraction

1. The cornea, lens, aqueous and vitreous.
2. Pupil constriction, convergence and accommodation.
3. For 'normal' eyesight.
4. Hypermetropia and myopia.
5. Astigmatism.
6. Diplopia.
7. Objective.
8. A sphere.
9. Astigmatism.
10. A prism.
11. To correct presbyopia.

Chapter 5

Preoperative cataract information

1. The lens begins to swell as the cataract develops, which alters the eye's refractive power.
2. Because the visual axis is involved.
3. A metabolic cataract.
4. Steroids.
5. Intumescent.
6. The focimeter.
7. Keratometry, lens power and axial length.
8. 23 mm.
9. Hypermetropic.

Chapter 6

Intraoperative management of cataract patients

1. The oculocardiac reflex or Aschner phenomenon.
2. Atropine.
3. Any two of these: subtenon's, retrobulbar, peribulbar or intracameral (if the patient experiences pain during surgery).
4. A topical approach. This is 'vocal' because the patient must be able to respond to the surgeon's instructions (to look at the microscope light, to keep their eye still and to not squeeze their eyelids shut).
5. Surgically induced pupil miosis.
6. To help prevent surgically induced pupil miosis.
7. Because (as well as wanting to monitor the patient's overall condition) there is a possibility that carbon dioxide will build up under the drapes if additional oxygen is not administered.
8. The surgeon.
9. A circular tear in the anterior lens capsule.
10. To mobilise the hard lens nucleus within the capsular bag.
11. To a 'dropped nucleus' into the vitreous or to vitreous getting into the anterior chamber.

Chapter 7

Postoperative cataract care

1. Acute pain and worsening vision in the operated eye.
2. Because lens implants have been re-designed to prevent the problem.
3. Because it is a danger both to eyesight and the structure of the eye. (Sometimes a cluster of cases occur whereby reasons for the outbreak must be discovered and preventive measures taken.)
4. Because the intraocular lens prescription often permits reasonable, unaided distance vision and spectacle correction may need to be adjusted.

5. Double vision. Patients can try covering one of their eyes. (The surgeon needs to be aware of the problem so that second eye surgery can be expedited.)

6. Because it can occur after complicated surgery, previous attacks, and infection.

7. Uveitis and because the patient is a steroid responder.

Chapter 8

The glaucomas, primary open-angle glaucoma and congenital glaucoma

1. 2%.

2. 10–21 mmHg.

3. The trabecular pathway and the uveoscleral pathway.

4. Examination of the optic disc, intraocular pressures and visual fields.

5. Yes, it is more common in black people.

6. Because they have thinner corneas.

7. The thickness of the cornea.

8. Any one of eyedrops, laser trabeculoplasty.

9. Generally with eye-drops because lowering the intraocular pressure by 30% is beneficial.

10. There are none until large areas of the visual field are lost.

Chapter 9

Primary angle-closure glaucoma

1. Hypermetropes.

2. Any two from hypermetropia, lens size, more anterior lens placement, a shallow anterior chamber, a small cornea and short axial length of the eye.

3. A 'warning' attack, which clears without treatment.

4. Any two from sudden, severe pain affecting the eye and brow, haloes around lights, a rapid fall in visual acuity and feeling poorly.

5. A crimson red conjunctiva, hazy cornea, discoloured iris or a fixed semi-dilated pupil.

6. Acetazolamide (Diamox™) 1 g in 24 hours.

7. Laser iridotomy.

8. No. (Research has shown the chances of this causing a problem are close to zero.)

Chapter 10

The secondary glaucomas

1. A phacolytic glaucoma or a phacomorphic glaucoma.

2. Any two of red cell glaucoma, ghost cell glaucoma and angle recession glaucoma.

3. Any two of haemorrhagic glaucoma, thrombotic glaucoma, congestive glaucoma, rubeotic glaucoma and diabetic haemorrhagic glaucoma.
4. Steroid responders.
5. An inflammatory glaucoma.
6. Pigment dispersal syndrome.
7. In women.

Chapter 11
Retinal problems

1. Any two from myopia, ageing, trauma and cataract surgery.
2. Any two from laser treatment, cryothermy and explant (plomb, encirclement, retinopexy, silicone tamponade, vitrectomy).
3. Retinopathy of prematurity.
4. It affects both.
5. Because the retina is in danger of 'peeling off' further. If the macula is still 'on' then the situation is more critical.
6. Because manipulating the extraocular muscles when placing the band causes increased discomfort and because the band itself is tight.
7. From blunt trauma to the eye.
8. Neovascular glaucoma.
9. Any two from smoking, cardiovascular disease, hypertension and hyperlipidaemia.

Chapter 12
Age-related macular degeneration

1. Any two from genetic factors, smoking, obesity, race, gender, diet and prolonged sun exposure.
2. Dry. It accounts for 90% of cases.
3. Any two from distortion of straight lines, subdued colour perception and reduced visual acuity.
4. Visual acuity tests such as the logMAR, Amsler test, near vision test, or the Ishihara colour test, RAPD or IOP.
5. OCT (ocular coherence tomography) and angiography.
6. To stop smoking, to reduce exposure to ultraviolet light, to improve their diet (and take vitamin supplements) and to cooperate with their GP in the control of hypertension and blood cholesterol.
7. Ranibizumab.
8. Sudden pain, a further reduction in visual acuity, floaters or flashing lights.

Index